SURVIVING
with
HEART

SURVIVING
with
HEART
TAKING CHARGE OF
YOUR HEART CARE

DARRELL TROUT & ELLEN WELCH

FOREWORDS BY NEIL R. BERCOW, M.D., AND SAMIN SHARMA, M.D.

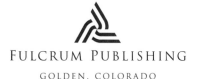

FULCRUM PUBLISHING

GOLDEN, COLORADO

We dedicate this book to all the exceptional heart patients who have taken charge
of their heart care and the caregivers who support them.

Library of Congress Cataloging-in-Publication Data

Trout, Darrell.
Surviving with heart : taking charge of your heart care /
Darrell Trout & Ellen Welch.
p. cm.
Includes bibliographical references and index.
ISBN 1-55591-201-X
1. Heart—Diseases—Popular works. I. Welch, Ellen. II. Title.
RC672 .T76 2002
616.1'2—dc21
2002008593

Printed in Canada
0 9 8 7 6 5 4 3 2 1

Editorial: Marlene Blessing, Ellen Wheat, Andrea Jarvela, Daniel Forrest-Bank
Design: Trina Stahl

Fulcrum Publishing
16100 Table Mountain Parkway, Suite 300
Golden, Colorado 80403
(800) 992-2908 • (303) 277-1623
www.fulcrum-books.com

CONTENTS

ACKNOWLEDGMENTS

WE WANT TO express our gratitude to Bob Baron, a publisher who continues to bring books to market based on their substance and merits rather than a stereotypical formula. Marlene Blessing is a dream editor—knowledgeable, supportive, and amazingly positive in the face of chaos and deadlines.

We also want to thank all those who have helped us in many different ways with this book. They include: Jenifer Alpers, John Bieber, Abby Jane Brody, Alan Cohen, Jimmy Dunn, Lloyd and Sue Elder, Susan Lanford, Gwen Lischke, DiAnn Lisica, Julius and Dottie McLaurin, Susan Merna, Marcy Miller, Arnold and Norma Norsworthy, Linda Niedert, Mike Petrikat, Dr. Stuart Polisner, Vern Powers, Cathy Self, James and Betty Thompson, Cheryl Van Hoof and the staff and participants at the Cardiac Rehabilitation Program at Rapides Regional Medical Center in Alexandria, Louisiana, Catherine Walker, and Marilyn Walker.

Darrell would like to express his individual gratitude to the following:
I want to thank all of the wonderful medical professionals who worked to save my life: Dr. Meyer Ballas, Dr. Neil R. Bercow, Dr. Marvin Leder, Dr. Samin Sharma, and the surgical teams, nurses, support staff, and patient educators at Mt. Sinai Hospital and St. Francis Hospital, The Heart Center®. I also am indebted to all of the helpful staff at the Cardiac Fitness and Rehabilitation Center of St. Francis Hospital, particularly Beth Ann Grady–Acker, my case

manager.

I also wish to thank two people who believed in me as a writer, Elvin McDonald and Cathy Wilkinson Barash. Each recognized something they valued in my work and helped me move forward: Elvin enjoyed something I wrote as an amateur and sent it on to a magazine, and Cathy had enough faith in me to have me write my first book and her first book as an editor.

My friends and family deserve thanks for their support during my battle with heart disease and for tolerating the life disruptions while writing this book. I also must single out Geri for her support, caring, and patience through it all.

Ellen would like to express her individual gratitude to the following:
I want to thank my parents, Grady and Myrtle Welch, who are a model of healthy living. Their example continues to inspire me and their support is a constant encouragement to me.

It is with gratitude that I express appreciation to special friends and to my children, whose patience and support helped me get through this writing project.

I also want to thank the individuals who took the time to share their journey with me. Their stories continue to impact my life just as they will impact the lives of every reader.

FOREWORD

by Neil R. Bercow, M.D.
Cardiothoracic Surgeon, St. Francis Hospital,
The Heart Center, Roslyn, New York

St. Francis Hospital has the third largest cardiac caseload in the United States. The Heart Center's coronary bypass surgery program is the only one in New York State with a risk-adjusted mortality rate significantly below the statewide average for all three-year periods analyzed by the New York State Department of Health (1989–1996).

SURGEONS DEVELOP AND perfect new techniques on an ongoing basis. At St. Francis Hospital, the Heart Center, we lead the way, now operating on beating hearts, without the necessity of using the heart-lung machine to maintain life-sustaining functions through minimally invasive openings in the chest cavity, or by using the newest techniques to repair valves. These advanced procedures enable the patient to heal much faster with fewer complications, which results in patients getting back to their lives much sooner than before. Beating heart surgery gives us new options for older and sicker patients; particularly those at high risk for cerebral or neurological vascular events.

Patients and caregivers need to carefully select a surgeon and hospital that fulfills their needs. *Surviving with Heart* describes how to do that. When Darrell needed bypass surgery, he considered his options. He spoke to several surgeons, a process he called "interviewing," though to me, it felt like a discussion with a knowledgeable patient about his case. Later, he told me that he liked how I analyzed his case and surgical needs. That gave him confidence and trust in me, something every patient should have with their surgeon and hospital. He also researched statistics, looking for a hospital that successfully completed a significant number of bypass surgeries each year, with low mortality, along with high patient satisfaction. *Surviving with Heart* describes the process of selecting doctors, surgeons, and a hospital; valuable guidance for patients and caregivers.

Surgeons often spend more time with patients when they are under anesthesia than fully awake. Our focus is the immediate need to correct a problem: fix a malfunctioning valve, open closed arteries before a damaging heart attack occurs, or install a pacemaker to bring the electrical signals to the heart back in sync.

Unfortunately, there is little time for the surgeon to work with patients to improve their lifestyles. Cardiac rehabilitation, like our program at the De Matteis Cardiac Fitness and Rehabilitation Center, where Darrell was a patient, provides an excellent beginning for heart patients. *Surviving with Heart* provides additional guidance and ongoing advice for patients and caregivers on what should be their new and improved lifestyle. It shows them how to truly take charge of their heart care.

Additionally, all patients should have close follow-up with their cardiologists or internists. Recent research and literature suggest that most, if not all, heart surgery patients should be on a low cholesterol diet, as well as a cholesterol-lowering medication.

FOREWORD

by Samin Sharma, M.D.
Director of Interventional Cardiology, Mount Sinai Hospital
and Director of Catheterization Laboratory, New York City, New York

In the most recent report issued by the New York State Department of Health comparing risk-adjusted mortality rates, Mount Sinai Hospital was designated the safest center in the state for patients undergoing angioplasty. Dr. Sharma achieved this highest level of safety and success for angioplasty by arriving at a less than two-tenths of one percent complication rate, while completing more than 1,000 of these procedures each year since 1997. He teaches at Mount Sinai School of Medicine where he received the Teacher of the Year Award in 2000.

IN RECENT YEARS, medical intervention techniques for the heart have seemingly become routine. As a team in the Catheterization Laboratory at Mount Sinai Hospital we have developed a system to open artery blockages in the safest way. We use percutaneous transluminal coronary angioplasty—balloon angioplasty—to open arteries clogged with a dangerous accumulation of fatty molecules and cholesterol called plaque. Angioplasty is a significant treatment of choice for many patients that restores normal blood flow to the heart. The cardiologist inserts a catheter—a narrow, hollow tube—into the patient's groin and carefully threads it through the artery, while monitoring with X-ray, to the blockage. A second, thinner catheter is inserted through the hollow tube.

Once positioned, a balloon on the end of the inner catheter is inflated, pushing against the artery-clogging plaque and widening the opening. Often a stent—a wire mesh tube—is inserted into the artery and helps prevent the plaque from closing the artery. We achieve success through the skilled use of these techniques and other devices. For example, to open particularly dense blockages, we use the rotoblator, a miniature, diamond-tipped high-speed drill (up to 60 times the speed of a car engine). I used this technique to open one of Darrell's blockages that had formed within a stent from a previous angioplasty.

In order to obtain optimal results, we need to thoroughly understand the overall health of the patient. Each patient is a unique case and needs to be treated accordingly. During the procedure, I monitor how the patient is doing, along with blood pressure and chest pain.

Prior to the procedure, it is important for the patient to develop trust in the doctor. Patient and doctor must be able to communicate well in order for this to happen. *Surviving with Heart* explains the heart and coronary artery disease in easily understood terms. It teaches patients how to describe their symptoms in order to communicate clearly with their doctors.

Through his struggles with heart disease, Darrell developed a good understanding of what was happening to his body. By his second angioplasty, he could accurately describe his symptoms and what he was experiencing. Thanks to this, we developed excellent communication and trust. He, along with his co-author Ellen Welch, has used that ability to help others in the same health crisis understand what is happening to them.

After angioplasty or bypass surgery, a patient must take charge of his or her life and heart care. The authors use Darrell's story and the stories of others to show you how to do it. They take you step-by-step through making such heart-healthy choices as eating right, exercising, reducing stress, quitting smoking—all choices that can help everyone stay healthy for years.

Patients need to seek out the best doctors and hospitals for heart care and form a partnership. *Surviving with Heart* provides a simple and complete roadmap for the patient with coronary artery disease to learn how to take charge of their heart care. Combining the best medical team and the information in *Surviving with Heart* will give patients the best odds of not only surviving, but thriving in the future.

A SPECIAL CAUTION TO READERS—PLEASE READ THIS

SURVIVING WITH HEART is intended to be reader-friendly by turning serious scientific studies and the latest research into readable text. It is meant to inspire patients to learn as much about heart disease, enabling such patients to be advocates for their well-being. The book is not a "do-it-yourself" guide and does not take the place of trained medical personnel, experienced cardiologists, and other specialists. It may help you determine when you need to see a doctor or seek emergency medical assistance. When in doubt, see a doctor or dial 911 if necessary. The book will better prepare you for your visit with a doctor and enable you to look out for your own interests. It will not replace medical diagnosis and care from a professional.

All books about medical topics have the following limitations:

Medical research constantly adds to our knowledge as new findings, techniques, and medications enter the marketplace. As SURVIVING WITH HEART goes into production, it reflects current understanding of heart disease and research from sources believed to be accurate. Patients and readers should always avail themselves of all current research and thinking and not use the book as a definitive source of information.

The explanation of complicated medical procedures, terms, and studies has been summarized and simplified to make the information understandable for individuals without medical training in a book of reasonable length rather than several volumes.

Every individual case of heart disease needs specific and personalized attention. A single book can never deal with the myriad of complex issues and problems every patient will face. Only trained physicians can evaluate and dispense effective advice on what treatment is needed by a patient.

The writers, reviewers, editors, and publisher are not engaged in providing medical services, and this book is not intended to diagnose or treat medical or physical problems.

This book is sold without warranties of any kind, express or implied, and the publishers, editors, and authors disclaim any liability, loss, or damage caused by the contents of this book.

Be careful in the use of this book. Always consult competent medical personnel for professional guidance.

INTRODUCTION

Starring Roles: Empowered Heart Patients and Caregivers

THE HEART IS the center of our beings. Matters of the heart govern our lives and our health. We write to you from our hearts because we care about you and your heart.

We did not begin our heart care education effort in order to write a book. We were looking for answers to critical health questions. "How do I stay alive with heart disease?" "How do I help my loved ones who have heart disease stay alive?" "How do I avoid future problems?" What follows are the answers to our questions—questions from Darrell, the heart patient, and Ellen, a caregiver, who has a family history of heart disease.

These personal answers have huge implications for a society battling an epidemic, an epidemic that to a great degree is preventable. American Heart Association (AHA) statistics show this leading killer of men and women in the United States claims the lives of 41.4 percent of the more than 2.3 million Americans who die each year. Coronary heart disease is the nation's leading killer. It takes the life of more than one victim every minute of every day—over 2,500 lives each day (calculated from AHA numbers)!

How can this continue to happen when we have had so many amazing discoveries from research? Surgical techniques get better every day, with the miracle of angioplasty and bypass operations opening the closed arteries of millions of individuals. With all of this progress why hasn't the epidemic been stopped in its tracks?

We believe the answer lies in the patients. They can control much of their own fate, become exceptional patients, and survive and thrive in the future. For years, people were taught that doctors were god-like and would cure you. They give you a magic pill or open your body and excise the disease. Today's doctors are far too busy to take complete control and responsibility for every patient's ongoing disease management. Prevention of heart disease and recovery is in large part up to the patient, with help from the best medical professionals.

In this book, we provide the background and tools to empower patients and caregivers to work as a team to fight the scourge of heart disease. We purposefully continue using the word *patient* all through the book, even for individuals who have recovered and thrived in spite of the disease. What these exceptional patients are doing is taking charge of their heart care and continuously fighting the battle because they know they are not cured. The opened artery from an angioplasty and the two, three, or more added arteries after bypass surgery do not cure anyone of heart disease. These invasive and sometimes dangerous procedures provide symptomatic relief from pain and may reduce the chance of dying from a heart attack, but they are not a cure. The underlying cause of clogged arteries (atherosclerosis) will continue closing them unless patients take charge and make changes. We give you that roadmap to a new journey through life.

For us, this is personal and not an academic writing exercise. We are motivated from first-hand experience. In August 1998, Ellen's seventy-four-year-old father underwent a quadruple bypass after experiencing two years of heart-related problems, including congestive heart failure. In October 1998, Darrell underwent triple bypass surgery after eleven months of problems, including a misdiagnosis and three angioplasties. Both Ellen's father and Darrell are diabetic and have high blood pressure. Our personal stories are woven throughout the book as are the stories of many additional heart patients and caregivers (most of their names are changed to protect their privacy). Their stories and ours will help you to understand the disease better and how we fight it. There are applicable quotes, from a wide range of sources, to interest you and help us make our points.

The massive numbers of deaths, a horror of the statistics, affect our nation and world. The pain, suffering, and death are personal; the afflicted are we, our friends, family, or loved ones. With over 43 percent of all deaths attributable to heart disease and as many as 75 percent of all adults at risk, virtually every family will be touched by this problem. The disease is never singular, always touching our loved ones, either through genetics or because they are thrust into a caregiver role. As it affects more than the person with heart disease, we have taken the unique approach of presenting information for both the patient and the caregiver, written with their individual and joint needs in mind. The design of the book reinforces our desire to help you understand the critical part your relationships play in the ongoing recovery process. Not only is it imperative that the patient take charge of his lifestyle management, but it is critical that care-givers learn how to work as part of a team. A caregiver must also maintain control of her own lifestyle without increasing negative impact on her life. While we celebrate our survival, we will emphasize how you choose to live your life. The choices not only affect your life expectancy but also powerfully influence the generations that follow.

We have created a concise six-point action plan that will inform and motivate you to become STAR patients and caregivers. As in any movie or stage production, the star is the central character. We give the patient and caregiver the starring roles—both are central to this effort. Each point adds support and knowledge for patients to create their own cohesive plan to battle heart disease and to achieve the best possible result, with some patients able to reverse the disease. We will help you create a positive patient–caregiver relationship. Most of us are surprised when we get sick or have to deal with a major crisis. Most individuals and families are not programmed to cope with the uncertainty of a life-threatening disease. Humans are optimistic by nature and often feel they will live forever. The reality of becoming a heart patient changes that very quickly. You are in a life-threatening situation. Caregivers face the potential loss of a loved one. Support is a significant key to surviving and thriving.

Through the STAR POINTS, the core of this book, we encourage readers to take charge of their bodies and heart care, and we show you how to do it.

We share our own stories and the experiences of other patients and caregivers. Our six-point plan includes:

STAR POINT ONE: Take Charge of Your Heart
STAR POINT TWO: Educate Yourself
STAR POINT THREE: Lead Your Team
STAR POINT FOUR: Manage Your Treatment
STAR POINT FIVE: Live Heart Smart
STAR POINT SIX: Embrace Support

In **STAR POINT ONE: Take Charge of Your Heart,** you learn the symptoms of heart disease and how to distinguish everyday aches and pains from life-threatening ones. Getting to the hospital in time is critical with a heart attack. Hundreds of thousands of lives are lost each year because individuals do not go to the hospital when they should. We also describe the risk factors for heart disease. We distinguish between the controllable ones and the others. You can affect cholesterol levels, diabetes, high blood pressure, obesity, stress, a high-fat diet, and a sedentary lifestyle, and, in some cases, totally avoid or control the problem.

In **STAR POINT TWO: Educate Yourself,** we emphasize that knowledge and understanding are powerful—a philosophy that runs throughout the book. You will learn about the amazing pumping machine, your heart, and how it keeps you alive. We show what can go wrong and some of the tests you might have. It all provides understanding for what's ahead and the ability to communicate with your medical team.

STAR POINT THREE: Lead Your Team demonstrates how to take charge or become part of the decision making. You learn how to select doctors, surgeons, and hospitals and how to work with them to get the best results.

STAR POINT FOUR: Manage Your Treatment gives you background to sort out the confusing issues of prescribed medications and types of surgery.

Powerful drugs can save your life but can also kill you if used improperly or in wrong combinations with other drugs, over-the-counter products, even with certain foods, herbs, and supplements. We provide suggestions to get control over your medical arsenal. We describe surgical procedures and discuss some of the benefits and risks.

We teach you to **Live Heart Smart** in **STAR POINT FIVE.** This is the lifestyle to lead in order to maintain a healthy life, or even to reverse heart disease. We guide you in cutting stress, eating a low-fat diet, controlling blood pressure and blood sugar, getting active, how to stop smoking, and finally, encourage you to take advantage of cardiac rehab.

STAR POINT SIX: Embrace Support looks at support systems and the mind–body relationship. We show you how to use and improve your support structures to help you survive. The power of the mind embraces spirituality, optimism, and passion as part of an engaged and positive life.

The final chapters of the book look at the impact of heart disease on women, children, and others in your life. You can and need to be an example for future generations that have the same genetic risks as you. Most people do not know that heart disease is the biggest killer of women in America. Women are ten times more likely to die of heart problems than breast cancer. We detail differences in symptoms and how a woman should demand and get better treatment. We also show how you can reach others and start to change the world "one person at a time."

What follows is about hope and celebrating life. If you are reading this, you or a loved one has a problem. We share our personal stories and guide you through the challenge of heart disease. We have survived, and we will teach you how to survive.

SECTION ONE

BECOME A STAR PATIENT *and* CAREGIVER

STAR POINT ONE

Take Charge of Your Heart

DARRELL'S STORY

"It took me a while to 'get it.' The miracles of modern medicine and the medicine men themselves were not going to wave their magic scalpels and catheters and make me well. The initial shock and confirmation of heart disease was mitigated several days later when my artery was opened by the magic of angioplasty. I figured I was done with the doctors; I was cured and could go back to my old life. Well, I was very wrong. I was not cured and I had to change my life if I were going to survive. That realization was the first huge step toward awareness, knowledge, and a healthy lifestyle. I think it always takes us time to absorb the reality of heart disease or any other major life-threatening disease. What's important is accepting that reality as a challenge and not accepting defeat. Allowing the negative to take over your life may not kill you—though some people think it can—but it certainly leaves you with no quality of life. I ultimately chose surgery to have a high quality of life—I would not settle. I also was determined to change my lifestyle in order to live. An oft-repeated saying is, 'It's not the years in your life that matters, it's the life in your years.' I choose to live—in order to do that, I have to be in charge. I don't think there is any other way.

"I feel lucky that I am attuned to my body. As my battle with heart disease continued, I became even more aware of what was happening to my body and inside my head. I think it is the only sensible way to approach the battle. You need some understanding of where you stand. The awareness of my body put me in a position to anticipate what would happen. Knowledge let me deal with it. The combination made me feel powerful and in charge and that helped me move forward rationally and recover more quickly."

AWARENESS AND KNOWLEDGE are crucial words for the patient's vocabulary. They empower the heart patient to move forward after surgery or a heart emergency. They also enable the caregiver to move forward. Caregivers who learn about heart disease and keep up with their patient's physical and emotional well-being offer the most help to their patient's ongoing recovery and healthy lifestyle. Learn to listen to your patient as your patient learns to listen to his or her body.

LISTEN TO YOUR BODY

THE FIRST STEP in taking charge of your health is learning to listen to your body. You can never describe something to a doctor if you don't know that it happened or you don't sense or feel it. Doctors working in the emergency room of busy Bellevue Hospital in New York City concluded that more than 60 percent of the diagnosis comes from *listening* to patients. That gives you some idea of how important it is to be able to know what is happening with your body and be able to describe it. For about one-third of people with heart disease the first symptom is a major heart attack. At least some of those individuals may have experienced small or minute changes or problems and simply ignored them. Men are notorious about not wanting to go to a doctor. Women must also learn to listen to their bodies and not ignore symptoms that frequently differ and are less obvious than men's. Those visits and regular checkups may save your life.

DARRELL'S STORY

"I was never sick with a major illness or spent a day in a hospital. I worked out, walked four miles most days, and had a decent diet. Then, bam, I was telling people about what my cardiologist said. Even just saying 'my cardiologist' was a shock."

Distinguish Between Minor Aches and Life-Threatening Pain

An important skill is to know when you should dial 911. If you are ever in a situation wondering if you should call 911—you should! Never take a chance. The odds are high that if you are having severe pain, difficulty breathing, light-headedness, sudden numbness of your leg(s), arm(s), or face, sudden trouble walking, dizziness, or a sudden severe headache, then dial 911 immediately—take no chances.

Do not drive yourself to the hospital; call an ambulance. You know that if you walk into an emergency room you are likely to sit there and wait while they attend to those "most in need of care." If you come in an ambulance, the EMS personnel will constantly monitor your vital signs on the trip and hospital personnel will move you directly into a cardiac care unit.

HEART POINT

DIAL 911 if you have: difficulty breathing, light-headedness, sudden numbness (of legs, arms, or face), sudden trouble walking, dizziness, or sudden severe headache.

DARRELL'S STORY

"It was Thanksgiving and I had consumed far too much food and wine. My brother-in-law, his wife, and kids were staying with us. We had just finished cleaning up the kitchen and dining room when the second-floor carbon monoxide detector screeched its warning. As I climbed the stairs to check the battery, pressure intensified in my back until it turned into pain. My 'back' was acting up again (I had gone to the doctor when I had 'back pain' and shooting symmetrical pain in my arms and wrists during my

HEART POINT

The American Heart Association, in its journal Circulation, recommends taking one 325-mg aspirin tablet at the first sign of a heart attack. They estimate that this will save over 10,000 lives each year. Those who take an aspirin have a 23 percent lower death rate and a reduced risk of stroke and of suffering another heart attack. (See more about daily use of aspirin in Star Point Four.)

four-mile health walk). The pain intensified until I could not reach up, remove the batteries, and shut the detector off. The screech continued as I moved to the bed to lie down. As I rested, the pain started to diminish. My wife came upstairs to see what was going on, and I told her about my 'back pain.' She removed the battery from the detector, and I rested until the pain went away. In the middle of the night I was awakened from a sound sleep by more 'back pain.' It got worse, and no matter how I moved, the pain pushed on my back and then intensified until I felt it through my entire chest cavity. After twenty minutes, though it seemed like hours, the pain disappeared entirely, and I collapsed back on the bed and slept. The next morning I called the doctor and went to his office. After describing these incidents, he gave me a shot of steroids for my 'back.' Though I did not have a heart attack I should have dialed 911 and gone to the hospital. At least I would have been diagnosed properly earlier in the process."

Self-Monitoring Skills

Every person should develop a heightened self-awareness of his or her body and become aware of how it works. Our heart beats, we breathe, our blood moves and is enriched with oxygen every minute of every day, and we don't think about it. We not only want you to think about it, we want you to become very aware of what your body typically feels like. Some individuals experience only vague symptoms prior to a heart attack. Being aware of your body and attuned to changes may save your life.

Your Breathing

Go into a quiet room and think about breathing. In fact, breathe audibly and listen to your breath sounds. Then do it less consciously but still monitor the air coming in and then going out. The more familiar you are with normal breathing, the easier it will be to know when and if breathing becomes "labored." Also, note the differences in breathing when you exercise. As you work harder, feel the changes and how your breathing increases to provide the higher levels of oxygen your body requires.

HEART POINT

A heart attack, or myocardial infarction, is a blockage of a coronary artery that cuts off the blood supply to a part of the heart. Heart tissue that is denied oxygen for periods of time dies.

Then note, as exercise continues, how breathing seems to stabilize. Note how your breathing returns to normal after any strenuous activity is completed.

Your Heartbeat

Most of the time, we are not aware of our heart beating. Perhaps only when you lift something heavy, exercise, or experience something scary or exciting do you note the increase in your heart rate, the number of heartbeats per minute. Spend a little time thinking about your heart. Monitor your heartbeat at rest, under stress, or during exercise, and notice the differences. You will learn what is normal or typical under varying conditions and be more aware of changes.

HEART POINT

Your heart rate is the number of times your heart beats during a specific time interval, usually measured in beats per minute.

LEARN THE SIGNIFICANCE OF SPECIFIC SYMPTOMS

Pressure or Pain in the Chest, Neck, and Arms

If you feel sudden excruciating pain in your chest, or sometimes in your back, particularly if it radiates into your shoulders or arms (or they tingle) and is accompanied by shortness of breath, sweating, or dizziness, it signals a serious medical emergency. If you have occasional pain or pressure or if it's brought on by exertion, stop what you are doing and see a doctor. Women often feel a burning sensation in their chest and may experience a tingling of arms and shoulders, and a general agitation or apprehension.

HEART POINT

Classic angina, or angina pectoris, is chest pain caused by inadequate blood flow (oxygen) to the heart muscle, caused by partially or totally blocked arteries.

Pain is a warning. The location of the pain(s), the severity, and the duration are important indicators of a problem and the magnitude of that problem. Is it a muscle pull, indigestion, a bruise, or angina? Heart problems and cardiovascular disease create different symptoms and pain(s) in different patients. Men and women differ in how their bodies respond to these problems.

Even a heart attack is not painful for all patients. We tend to picture a man shoveling heavy, wet snow suddenly dropping the shovel and clutching his chest in excruciating pain. Some patients describe chest pain with additional pain radiating down both arms to the fingertips, particularly the left hand, along with shortness of breath. That level of pain needs an immediate response—dial 911 and get yourself to the hospital.

JOHAN'S STORY
(heart patient, 55)

"I had a heart attack and was in the hospital. They used angioplasty and opened my left anterior descending artery that was 99 percent closed. In the middle of the night I had incredible pain. The medical team gathered around my bed and asked me to describe the pain. I told them that I couldn't. The doctor then said to me, 'You'd better learn or we will open you up.' I then described a specific pain going across my chest, which must have been very different from heart attack pain. They did not take me into surgery; I stabilized and was fine in the morning."

Pain is sometimes difficult to describe; sometimes it's even difficult to know where it comes from in the body. We've all had a toothache and were surprised to find out that a tooth other than the one we thought was the problem was, in fact, the problem. Any substantial pain that lasts for more than a few minutes should be checked out immediately at the hospital.

Women should be particularly concerned about any chest discomfort accompanied by shortness of breath. Most women do not think they are at risk for heart disease—they are dangerously wrong. Heart disease is the leading killer among women. It is also a sad truth that many physicians do not consider heart disease or a heart attack when a woman presents with these symptoms.

Pain with Exertion or Stress

Often the first warnings of heart disease occur during exercise or when you are doing heavy physical work. It can happen when you are shoveling snow, having sex, jogging, walking (especially uphill), or changing a flat tire on your car. Stress from an argument, on the job, or even wonderful events, like a wedding or holiday gathering of friends and family, can bring on this kind of pain. Any physical activity or stress that makes the heart work harder could result in pain.

ERNIE'S STORY
(heart patient, 54, as told by his brother Johan)

"Ernie was aware of his heart problems. Our mother had died of a heart attack. He was being treated with medication. I think that Ernie had symptoms for several days before his heart attack. Three days before, he told me that he was very tired. On a Saturday, while working on a house in Pennsylvania, he had chest pains, yet drove back to New York. On Sunday, he had chest pains again but would not let his wife call for an ambulance. That evening he had a heart attack, was taken to the hospital but never came out of it. He was only fifty-four but in denial. I do not want anyone to ignore symptoms like he did. Act on them; it can save your life."

Classic angina is thought of as chest pain that radiates throughout the chest, then into the back, neck, shoulders, and into the arms, particularly the left arm or left side of the body. Some patients have pain(s) that starts in areas other than the chest. Occasionally patients visit their dentists complaining of pain in their jaw when, in fact, the culprit is heart disease and angina.

DARRELL'S STORY

"It was a beautiful fall day. I was enjoying my health walk, watching the birds and the people in the park. I had covered about two miles when suddenly I had sharp, though not major, pains in both wrists simultaneously. I slowed, then picked up my pace again, only to have the pains return. I stopped and monitored my body for a few minutes and tried to figure out what was happening. I felt good, and the pain disappeared. I started walking, albeit a bit slower than before, and finished my four-mile walk. A few days later I mentioned the episode to my wife. She was concerned and said, 'I don't like the sound of that!' I said I felt fine and it must be nothing, I'm okay now. It was a few weeks before any pain returned. The pain was still localized in my wrists, but it went a bit farther up my arms this time. This time I made the first of many appointments over several months with my primary care doctor."

Duration of Pain

The duration of the pain is an important factor. A "twitch" of pain or very short duration pain usually is not considered angina. Angina occurs when there is not enough blood supply to fill the heart's need for oxygen. It usually lasts for several minutes. Any angina type pain that lasts for more than five minutes requires immediate medical care—call 911.

ALEX'S STORY
(heart patient, 55)

"I was working twelve stressful hours a day as an executive vice president for a company that was failing. I was miserable, worrying, very unhappy, yet trying to make it work. I awoke one Sunday evening shortly after going to sleep with pain in my throat (doctors later called it 'the necktie effect'). I had to sit up because it was too painful to lie down, and I also had major indigestion, including gas and bloating. I'm a nice Jewish kid who doesn't deal well with pain, so I took three aspirin (that saved me from heart damage). I stayed up all night being miserable with nothing else to do but smoke cigarettes and drink cognac. I did some research on the Internet and finally called my doctor on Tuesday and went to the hospital that night. After being in the hospital awhile I asked them, 'So, why am I here?' They said, 'You had a heart attack.'"

Other Discomfort

Rather than pain, a person might experience uncomfortable pressure, squeezing, or a feeling of fullness in the chest. Pain or discomfort might be in the back, neck, jaw, or stomach. "Really bad" indigestion can also be a symptom of a heart attack.

Shortness of Breath and Other Symptoms

A doctor should evaluate any shortness of breath that reoccurs or is persistent. If your shortness of breath has occurred suddenly, is severe, and is accompanied by chest pain, this is a medical emergency and you should call 911. Even without the chest pain, if the shortness of breath is severe, you should consider this an emergency.

Other symptoms may include light-headedness, nausea, or breaking out in a cold sweat.

Women may experience an overriding feeling of unease that may or may not be accompanied by any of the other just-mentioned symptoms.

Symptoms of a Stroke

Closed arteries may also cause a stroke, rather than a heart attack. Be aware of the following symptoms of a stroke and get emergency medical treatment:

♦ Sudden changes in vision
♦ Sudden weakness in arm, leg, or face
♦ Sudden, severe headache without a known cause
♦ Sudden change in your ability to understand speech or to speak
♦ Difficulty standing, unsteadiness, or unexplained dizziness
♦ Drowsiness, nausea, or vomiting

KNOW WHAT TO DO IN AN EMERGENCY

LIVING WITH HEART disease can mean several trips to the hospital. If you know what to do in a heart emergency situation you will feel more empowered.

HEART POINT

Forty percent of the 1.1 million heart attacks in the United States each year are fatal. Only one in five patients gets to the emergency room early enough to benefit from life-saving treatments that break up blood clots in the arteries that cause damage to the heart.

If the patient, caregiver, and their family and friends have a plan in place, then everyone will feel more at ease. Call the nearest local fire station to ask paramedics how long it would take them to get to the patient's house or apartment and alert them to the patient's condition. Find out if an emergency vehicle would come from the fire station or a hospital.

If the caregiver does not live with the patient, decide on a regular time to call each other weekly. If a heart attack or surgery has taken place, you might want to check in nightly or each morning for several months. If each of you has e-mail, a daily e-mail report from the patient could replace a phone call.

Many caregivers who do not live with their patients fear that something will happen and the patient will not be able to get help. Finding a trusted neighbor or friend who will physically go by and check on your patient can calm your fears. There are also emergency signaling devices a patient can have on his or her body to summon help immediately in case of a problem.

DANIEL'S STORY
(caregiver, 38)

"My dad has nearly died several times. He has had some close calls at home. Either my wife or I started calling or going over to check on him every day. I have a house key, so if he doesn't answer the phone or the door, I will not hesitate to go in and check on him. I know that my dad doesn't tell me every time he has chest pains, so keeping a close check on him and watching for any changes in his behavior or health eases my mind."

Emergency Planning

Having an emergency plan is important—whether you are a patient or caregiver. In addition to knowing when to call 911 or go to the hospital, what are other ways in which you should be prepared for medical emergencies?

Post important phone numbers for the following agencies next to your telephone or in a conspicuous place where they can easily be seen by anyone. For example:

- Physician's name and number (emergency and office number)
- Hospital name and number
- Home health agency/nurse, if one is currently making visits to the home
- Telephone numbers where caregiver can be reached
- Neighbors' names and phone numbers
- Names and phone numbers of nearby relatives
- Name and phone number of a minister

Be sure certain substitute caregivers know important numbers and any special information about the patient. Give substitute caregivers a list of the patient's medications in case of an emergency in your absence.

Call the Doctor

If you are a caregiver for a person with heart disease, there are additional symptoms that are important to know. Keep the doctor's phone number by your phone, bedside, and in your purse or billfold. Call the doctor immediately if you notice any of the following symptoms in your patient:

- A feeling of fullness or bloating in the stomach with a loss of appetite or nausea
- Extreme fatigue or decreased ability to complete daily routines and activities
- A respiratory infection or a cough that becomes worse
- Constant dizziness or light-headedness
- New, irregular heartbeat
- Chest pain or discomfort brought on by activity and relieved when resting
- Difficulty breathing during regular activity or at rest
- Changes in sleep patterns
- Decreased urination
- Restlessness, confusion

CARDIOPULMONARY RESUSCITATION (CPR)

If a person stops breathing or the heart stops beating, permanent brain damage or death will occur if breathing and circulation functions are not quickly restored. CPR keeps the heart and circulation going until help arrives, and that can save a life. The American Red Cross regularly teaches CPR courses. In addition, it is often taught at community centers, community colleges, churches, fire stations, and sometimes schools. Completing a CPR course will give you a feeling of confidence that you can help your patient survive if an emergency arises.

Why Don't People Get Help?

Some heart patients will ignore symptoms, putting themselves at further risk. They don't want to cause additional problems. Some want to stay in denial that anything could be wrong. Others are afraid of the potential medical procedures their condition might require.

Caregivers should know that no matter what the patient's excuse, if you feel the patient needs help, get it. If you think the situation could be serious and your patient refuses to go to the doctor or the hospital, call 911 anyway. Explain to your patient, "I understand that it is your body, but because I love you and care about you, I am calling for help. I could not handle it if something happened to you because we did not get help."

JOHAN'S STORY
(heart patient, 55)

"After my heart attack and angioplasty, my wife and daughter wanted to be better prepared for another emergency. They both completed a CPR course. They felt more in control and better able to handle emergencies. It made me feel better also."

KNOW YOUR HEART DISEASE RISK FACTORS

"I will kill thee a hundred and fifty ways."
—WILLIAM SHAKESPEARE (1564–1616), *As You Like It* (ACT 5, SCENE 1)

EVERYONE NEEDS TO understand the underlying risk factors for heart disease. Some factors—age, sex, and family history—are out of our control. You can influence or totally control some risks by making the correct lifestyle choices. Research from the Centers for Disease Control and Prevention determined how the following factors relate to an individual's general health:

1. lifestyle—53%
2. environment—19%
3. heredity—18%
4. quality of medical care—10%

Knowing the importance of each of the heart disease risk factors will help you make the best decisions. Your lifestyle choices are the largest contributing factor to your health. Wise choices can add years to your life or even save your life. It's also important to know that having several risk factors multiplies your risk of having heart disease.

Family History

The genes you inherited from your parents, who, in turn, inherited them from their parents, have a significant impact on your health. When you first visit a doctor, you are asked many questions about your health history and your blood relatives. There are numerous studies that show that if coronary heart disease is common in families before the age of fifty-five, you are much more likely to experience an early heart attack.

DARRELL'S STORY

"After my first angioplasty I started talking to my family about others who have had heart disease. I was surprised to learn that both of my grandfathers had died of some form of heart disease. My paternal grandfather died at fifty-five, and my maternal grandfather died of a heart attack at the age of sixty-three. I also started hearing about high blood pressure, diabetes, and other problems in my family. I was aware of relatives dying young, I just was not aware of the full history."

There is important information in your own family history. If someone has already done research and created a family tree, you are well on your way to creating a major information device for you and your doctors. It can also work as an early warning system. Your family's medical history can predict threats of serious disease and death. This document will also prove valuable to your children and their children.

Creating a Family Medical History
Start by collecting the basic information that you need for a family tree: names and birth and death dates for parents, grandparents, and all offspring. Collect as much information as you can on all serious illness and disease and the dates of occurrence. For example, you would want to record that Grandpa Charley had a heart attack in 1952 and that he recovered and lived another thirty years. Record any information about strokes, high blood pressure, and diabetes. If a death was unexplained, note that, particularly if it was a sudden death. Do the same for living relatives, paying particular attention to any heart or vascular problems and surgeries (bypass surgery or balloon angioplasty). Determine if any of those relatives are taking medications for elevated cholesterol or triglycerides, high blood pressure, or coronary heart disease (such as nitroglycerine to relieve the pain and pressure of angina). Indicate those who smoked plus any environmental hazards they faced.

Create a large chart to show this information; it makes it easier to see the whole history before your eyes. Start with grandparents at the top of the chart, with their children directly below them. Chart all of your blood relatives, including aunts and uncles along with their children. With this information, you and your doctors are much better equipped to anticipate problems in your future.

It is important to gather as much data as possible. If you have only a few known blood relatives, work closely with them. Share all the information known and continue to update in future years.

If you have no data or known blood relatives, you need to be vigilant in watching for any changes and signs of disease in your body. There are genetic tests available to screen for the likelihood of developing certain health problems. Most of these tests, including those for several types of heart problems, are very involved and costly.

Age and Gender

Men over the age of forty-five, postmenopausal women, and women over fifty-five tend to be at the greatest risk of heart disease.

Smoking

There is massive evidence that smoking is detrimental to your health. Smoking alone produces a high incidence of heart disease along with many cancers. Secondhand smoke also harms those around you. In 1979, the Surgeon General examined over 30,000 studies and concluded in *Smoking and Health* that smoking is not only a major factor in death and disability but one of the worst health hazards in the United States. It is the primary cause of emphysema; is implicated in high blood pressure and chronic bronchitis; and is a factor in cancers of the lung, bladder, esophagus, larynx, kidney, mouth, pancreas, and stomach.

HEART POINT

The important result of quitting smoking is that within a few years, a former smoker's risk of a heart attack becomes virtually the same as that of a nonsmoker.

Even with all this evidence, over 26 percent of men and 21 percent of women over the age of eighteen in the United States smoke. The Centers for Disease Control and Prevention (CDCP) estimate that smoking and tobacco use result in over 400,000 deaths annually. In an even more astounding number, the CDCP estimates 100 million Chinese males now age twenty-nine or younger will die from smoking-related causes.

Smoking produces physical changes in your body. The first obvious sign is the speeding up of your heartbeat. Many smokers can feel the "hit" from the drugs in cigarettes. The walls of your blood vessels narrow and are damaged. The damaged locations are where plaque collects and narrows the opening. Oxygen going to the heart is reduced, and carbon monoxide replaces the oxygen. Your risk of heart disease or a heart attack increases more if you are a smoker with high blood pressure (hypertension) and elevated cholesterol.

A smoker's high-density lipoprotein (HDL), the so-called good cholesterol, will be lower than for a nonsmoker.

High Blood Pressure (Hypertension)

Blood pressure is the measure of the pressure of blood pumping through our arteries. Blood pressure is expressed as two numbers, for example 120/80. In this example, 120 is the systolic pressure, the measure of pressure when the heart beats. The other number, 80, is the diastolic pressure, the pressure when the heart rests. High blood pressure, technically called hypertension, is a higher-than-normal blood pressure. High blood pressure is defined as a systolic pressure of 140 mm Hg (mercury) or higher and a diastolic blood pressure of 90 mm Hg or higher.

HEART POINT

Hypertension is blood pressure that is measured as being 140 mm Hg or higher for systolic and 90 mm Hg or higher for diastolic.

The third National Health and Nutrition Examination Survey (NHANES III), from 1991–1994, estimates that approximately 23 percent of adults aged eighteen to seventy-four years have high blood pressure. As people age, the prevalence of high blood pressure increases. Despite how widespread it is, the NHANES III data indicate that 35 percent of those with high blood pressure don't know they have the condition.

The U.S. Department of Health & Human Services reports that an estimated 43 million Americans, including a greater percentage of older adults and African Americans, have high blood pressure. Experts now suggest that the objective of treatment should be to lower their blood pressure readings to 130–135/80–85 mm Hg, at least.

High blood pressure makes the heart work harder and may ultimately cause it to weaken or enlarge. If not controlled, it can lead to a stroke, heart attack, kidney failure, and damage to the eyes. Your risk of cardio-

HEART POINT

Hypertension was thought to be a disease of business executives. It is a disease of people in all types of jobs, including working mom and homemaker.

vascular disease increases tenfold if you smoke or have a high cholesterol level along with high blood pressure. Additionally disturbing is that only about 27 percent of those diagnosed with high blood pressure actually control it to suggested levels. The Framingham Heart Study shows that even relatively small elevations of blood pressure are dangerous. You have five times the risk of a heart attack if your diastolic blood pressure is between 85 and 94.

High blood pressure is often called a "silent killer" because people can walk around with it for years with no apparent symptoms while it continues to adversely affect their body. Everyone should have their blood pressure screened regularly by their doctor. If you have other heart disease risk factors or a family history of high blood pressure, start monitoring it early.

Your blood pressure should be measured at several different doctor visits and several different ways: sitting, standing, left and right arms. Readings can vary dramatically at different visits and times of day, so you need a series of readings before concluding that you have high blood pressure. Some patients also suffer from what is called "white-coat hypertension"—their blood pressures are elevated just by being in the doctor's office.

DARRELL'S STORY

"I have had high blood pressure and have been taking medication for more than five years. With medication, diet, and exercise my readings average 135/85. Recently, my endocrinologist has been fine-tuning medications to control it more tightly, aiming for as close to 120/80 as possible. I think the guidelines and definitions will soon change to reflect the research. Doctors will work to get everyone's blood pressure close to that level of control."

Diabetes

Diabetes mellitus is a medical condition in which the body is not able to produce enough insulin or the insulin the body makes does not work properly to process sugary or starchy foods.

The most common test for diabetes is a fasting glucose (a form of sugar; our bodies turn most food into sugar) blood test. You go for eight to ten hours without food before the nurse draws blood for the test. If the fasting blood sugar test indicates that there is 126 mg/dl (milligrams of glucose per deciliter of blood) or more of sugar present, a diagnosis of diabetes is made.

Diabetes is a progressive disease, and long-term uncontrolled diabetes—high blood sugar—can lead to very serious problems. The excess sugar affects all of the blood vessels of the body, which ultimately harms the heart and other organs. It also can lead to heart attack and stroke, sexual dysfunction, retinopathy (eye problems), kidney problems, neuropathy (nerve problems, which may include a loss of sensation or stabbing pains), foot problems, and gum disease. These can precipitate other major health crises such as blindness and amputation.

DIABETES WARNING SIGNS

1. Constant thirst or hunger
2. Frequent urination, day or night
3. Frequent skin infections
4. Blurred vision
5. Numb or tingling extremities
6. Slow healing of cuts and bruises
7. Fatigue and sleepiness
8. Unexplained weight loss

In recent years, the number of patients with diabetes has increased at alarming rates. There are two types of diabetes. Type I diabetes (formerly called juvenile onset diabetes) is generally diagnosed before the age of twenty. It is also sometimes referred to as insulin-dependent diabetes as patients are dependent on prescribed insulin. Type II diabetes (sometimes called adult onset or non-insulin-dependent diabetes) was generally diagnosed between the ages of forty and sixty. Now children as young as ten have this disease. A steady diet of fast food and sugary sodas and lack of exercise are major contributors to this growing epidemic. Diabetes at a young age can add untold misery later in life. Type II diabetes has a genetic component and is frequently passed from generation to generation, with the likelihood increasing as a person ages. If a person is overweight, or obese, that person is more likely to develop diabetes.

From 1990 to 1998 the number of patients with Type II diabetes jumped 33 percent overall, with an epidemic-like increase of 70 percent for individuals in their thirties. Sixteen million people in the United States are now diagnosed with diabetes.

The American Diabetes Association (ADA) revised its diabetes threshold guidelines in 1997 to a fasting glucose level of 126 mg/dl from 140 mg/dl. Diabetes research showed that complications from diabetes start much earlier than previously believed and can be avoided through good control of the disease. A patient can never be cured of diabetes, but he or she can control it.

HEART POINT

A diabetic's medical-care costs—$10,000 to $12,000 per year—are three to four times higher than those of healthy people.

With the new threshold, the ADA also hopes to identify an additional 2 million persons out of the 8 million believed to have the disease but who remain undiagnosed. Individuals with fasting glucose results of 110 mg/dl to 125 mg/dl are considered glucose impaired and are in danger of developing diabetes. They should be tested frequently and modify their lifestyle to avoid the disease. Eating a diet low in meat and dairy products, exercising, and keeping your weight down will help you avoid diabetes.

DARRELL'S STORY

"About three years before my diagnosis of heart disease, my fasting glucose levels started edging higher. My tests were coming back from the laboratories showing 135 mg/dl to 145 mg/dl. (The recognized threshold for an official diagnosis of diabetes was a fasting blood glucose level of 140 mg/dl and over.) My primary care physician said we should continue to monitor the levels and consider diabetes treatment, which I resisted. There was no education about diabetes, and I did no research. After my heart disease was diagnosed, I changed doctors. My new primary care physician is an endocrinologist who referred to my disease as an insidious form of diabetes. We both work hard to keep my blood sugars under control and to avoid complications."

Cholesterol: The Good, The Bad, and The Ugly

The National Heart, Lung, and Blood Institute describes high blood cholesterol as a serious problem and significant risk factor for heart disease.

The two major types of cholesterol are the low-density lipoproteins (LDL) and the high-density lipoproteins (HDL). An easy device for remembering which type is bad and which is good is to think of the LDL cholesterol as the "lousy" cholesterol, as it causes the cholesterol to build up or collect along your artery walls and begin to choke off blood flow. The HDL cholesterol helps remove cholesterol from your body and can be thought of as the "healthy" cholesterol.

Our bodies actually make cholesterol for use in necessary bodily functions. Problems occur when the body produces more cholesterol than required or we consume an excess of foods high in saturated fat or cholesterol. Saturated fat is the most significant factor in determining how much cholesterol your body creates. The cholesterol then moves with the blood but won't dissolve into it. The greater the quantity of it in the blood, the more likely it will collect on the artery walls—like sediment collecting in a drainpipe.

For the general population, total cholesterol readings over 240 mg/dl are considered high, 200–239 mg/dl borderline, and under 200 mg/dl a desirable level. If you have other heart disease risk factors, you and your doctor should attempt to lower your total cholesterol even more.

LDL levels should be under 160 mg/dl for the general population. If you have other risk factors, your target LDL level should be under 130 mg/dl. For those diagnosed with heart disease, desirable target level drops to 100 mg/dl or less.

The opposite is true for HDL cholesterol; raising it will decrease your risk of heart disease. An HDL level of less than 40 mg/dl is considered low, and 60 mg/dl is a good, protective-level reading. The HDL cholesterol helps "clean out the bad" LDL cholesterol.

The ratio of total cholesterol divided by HDL is also an important indicator. If the ratio is greater than 4, individuals should take action even if other indicators are in the acceptable range. If your HDL is 40, LDL 160, and total cholesterol 200, your ratio would be 5.0 (200/40).

Triglycerides

Triglycerides are the principal fats or lipids—a mixture of fatty acids and glycerol—circulating in the blood. The triglyceride level is an important factor in calculating your LDL level and can only be accurately measured after a 10- to 12-hour fast. Though studies have had mixed results, evidence is now suggesting that high levels of triglyceride are associated with an increased risk for heart disease. Although triglycerides do not collect in your arteries as LDL cholesterol does, they cause the blood to thicken, making clots more likely to form, and may also prevent the arteries from dilating to improve flow when needed. A desirable level (all measured in mg/dl) is less than 150, borderline high levels are between 150 and 199, and high levels are between 200 and 500, with very high readings above that.

Homocysteine

When your body's cells metabolize proteins, they create the amino acid homocysteine. Studies show that an elevated level of homocysteine is a risk factor for heart disease. There is still much to learn about homocysteine and how it adversely affects our bodies and arteries. There is no definitive level that triggers treatment. Dr. William P. Castelli, a former director of the Framingham Heart Study, suggests patients with levels greater than 10 micromoles per liter need treatment. For most people with normal homocysteine levels, simply eating foods rich in folic acid, such as spinach, orange juice, and beets, will prevent increasing levels. As an alternative, supplement your diet with a multivitamin that includes 400 micrograms per day of folic acid, or a separate folic acid supplement at that level.

Physical Inactivity

The heart is a muscle: one no bigger than your fist and one that many doctors would suggest is the most important muscle in your body. It, like other muscles in your body, needs exercise in order to stay strong and healthy. Heart exer-cises are called cardiovascular or aerobic. They raise the heart rate sufficiently to work the heart hard enough to improve its condition. Exercise has a number of benefits, including helping you control your weight. It has been shown to improve your level of HDL, the good choles-terol. Exercise improves your mood, and there are recent studies that show that exer-cise helps mental functioning in older adults. Numerous studies suggest that inactive peo-ple have a higher risk of a heart attack than those who get regular exercise.

HEART POINT

Body mass index (BMI) is determined by dividing weight in kilograms (one kilogram=2.2 pounds) by height in meters squared (one meter=39.37 inches).

Obesity

Excess weight and body fat put tremendous strain on the heart and other parts of your body. They also interrelate with several other heart disease risk factors. Losing weight has a positive effect on blood pressure, diabetes, cholesterol, and more. According to a study reported in the February 24, 2000, issue of *Diabetes Care* magazine, obese young adults are becoming diabetics at an earlier age than previously predicted. These patients also seem to have a higher incidence of high blood pressure and unhealthy blood lipid profiles. The study authors sug-gest that the *earlier onset of diabetes will lead to early heart disease.* Obesity alone adds to your heart disease risk and, when combined with the other risk factors, multiplies your risk.

The incidence of obesity is increasing at an alarming rate. Obesity is defined as being more than 30 percent over your ideal weight. Another indica-tor is body mass index (BMI). A healthy BMI ranges from 19 to 25. A BMI above 29 can be an independent risk factor for heart and other diseases. A BMI of 25–30 also increases your risk of heart disease if you also have other risk factors such as high blood pressure, smoking, diabetes, or high cholestrol. A National Center for Health Statistics report determined that 49 percent of women and 59 percent of men in the United States have a BMI over 25. Individuals between fifty and sixty years of age are even less healthy, with 64 percent of women and 73 percent of men labeled overweight or obese.

High-Fat Diet

The American Heart Association recommends that all Americans adopt a sensible diet high in fruits and vegetables and low in fat and cholesterol, particularly saturated fats.

The American high-fat diet is killing us. Landmark studies during World War II clearly demonstrated that, in Finland, when the population lived without meat, cheese, dairy, and other high-fat foods, the number of heart attacks reduced by two-thirds. In Japan, the standard diet—low in meat and dairy consumption, high in fish and vegetables—produces a low level of heart disease. When Japanese individuals immigrate to America and adopt our high-fat ways, they start to die of heart disease at the same rate we do.

> "The American high-fat diet is killing us."

Stress

"The mind is its own place, and in itself
Can make a Heav'n of Hell, a Hell of Heav'n."
—JOHN MILTON, *Paradise Lost* (1667)

Stress has always been controversial when considered as a cause of any disease. Most people have heard of the Type A person and behavior. The Type A phenomenon was described by Dr. Meyer Friedman in his book *Type A Behavior and Your Heart*. He described Type As as highly competitive, never having enough time, and trying to do many things at once. Frustrations associated with that behavior lead to anger. Anger produces real changes in our bodies. It can affect heart rate, respiration, muscle tension, and blood pressure. If someone is chronically stressed, those changes can lead to illness.

Dr. Dean Ornish's book *Dr. Dean Ornish's Program for Reversing Heart Disease* details his complete program. Dr. Ornish's research, described in his books and journal articles, shows that most of the patients who strictly follow his program reverse heart disease and have some symptomatic improvement. Stress reduction is one essential component of his research and program. A low-fat vegetarian diet and exercise are other parts of the approach.

Reducing stress in our lives leads to a more positive attitude and a happier existence. It helps us avoid other physical problems and destructive behaviors, including drinking, overeating and eating high-fat foods, smoking, and skipping exercise. These behaviors negatively affect most of the other risk factors.

UNDERSTAND THE CAREGIVER'S EMOTIONAL REACTIONS

ELLEN'S STORY

"I was used to hearing about people having heart attacks or bypass surgery. I guess I really didn't think too much about it. I thought because I heard about it so much that it was common and not a big deal anymore. But the day it became my father with heart disease and my father having bypass surgery, life completely changed. Suddenly, I took nothing about the medical technology for granted, and I haven't since the day I found out he was going to need surgery. At first, my concerns were just for my father and his condition; then as I researched more and found out that I, too, was at risk, it became even more personal—I am at risk and so are my children and their children. I also learned, thank goodness, that we can 'fight back' by taking control of our health. I became motivated to take the 'fight' to anyone and everyone."

"To thine own self be true."

—WILLIAM SHAKESPEARE (1564–1616), *Hamlet* (ACT I, SCENE 3)

HEART DISEASE IS a family affair. It attacks all kinds of families: young, old, rich, poor, weak, and strong. It creates all kinds of caregivers: daughters, sons, partners, spouses, parents, and friends. A life-threatening illness affects every person whose life intersects in any way with the patient. For the first months after the heart attack or heart surgery, the patient's well-being consumes the minds and emotions of those who care about the patient. It is easy to become overwhelmed with all the medical jargon and procedures and with all the doctor visits.

HEART POINT

A report from the National Caregivers Association estimates that there are 25 million people in America who find themselves in a caregiving role.

You have two equally important goals as a caregiver: (1) to do everything you can to take care of yourself so you are healthy and can support your patient, and (2) to encourage your patient to lead a healthy lifestyle. Although, as a caregiver, you are providing care and support, know that you cannot control your patient. The only person you can control is *you*. Before we start to educate you on anything related to heart disease and your patient, it is critical that we educate you on how to take care of yourself.

> "The best way to take care of your patient is to take care of yourself."

You know the speech that flight attendants give. They tell you that if the pressure inside the plane drops and you are seated next to a child or someone who needs assistance, put your oxygen mask on first before assisting someone else. Why? Obviously, if you are not conscious, you cannot help the person sitting beside you.

A caregiver is in a vulnerable position. Caregivers seldom understand that they are the only ones in the "heart disease process" who are in danger of sacrificing themselves while taking care of the patient. When your patient is recovering from surgery or is incapacitated for a period, you will have to be caretaker. However, when your patient starts recovering, you must move from caretaker to caregiver and help the patient learn to take care of his or her own health. You can help to motivate and change habits, but you cannot control your patient's behavior. It is crucially important that as a long-term caregiver you become as emotionally, mentally, physically, and spiritually healthy as possible. The best way to take care of your patient is to take care of yourself.

ELLEN'S STORY

"No one in our family knew how my father's surgery would affect us. When we stood in the ICU for the first time after his bypass surgery and saw him lying in the bed hooked up to machines, we lost it. Three generations stood there crying and looking at our patriarch, who was completely helpless. When you see someone who has done so much for you in a totally helpless position, you know that you will do anything to help them get better."

Our personalities and background influence how we deal with traumatic situations. In *The Complete Bedside Companion,* authors Philip Bashe and Rodger McFarlane suggest that caregivers respond to illness in character, just as patients do. Super-mom types may think they know more than the doctors, while passive–aggressive persons will start wringing their hands. If you are the dramatic type, then you will probably be an emotional extrovert during a heart emergency. If you are the quiet type, you will probably "shut down" even more and long for all the relatives and company to leave so you can be alone and take care of your patient. There really is no right or wrong way for you to react to a sudden heart emergency when it involves someone you love. But as soon as your patient starts to recover, so must you.

> "Learning to cope with a loved one's lifelong illness is a process."

The Lifelong Reality

The primary intent of this section is for you to understand the obstacles and challenges you face as you continue in your role as caregiver. Learning to cope with a loved one's lifelong illness is a process. The more experience you have with coping, the more opportunities you will have to understand yourself and to learn how to take care of yourself while caring for and about your patient.

For the first few weeks, months, and sometimes years following your patient's diagnosis, both you and your patient will work through the grief process. Usually we think about grief when someone dies, but we also grieve whenever we feel loss. Most transitions create some sense of loss, even good ones. When a family celebrates the birth of a baby, the parents and other siblings must let go of the normal routines they had before the baby: siblings may not get as much attention, and parents will lose sleep. Transitions such as divorce, job change, and moving all create some sense of leaving one life stage and moving on to a new one.

When your loved one suffered a heart attack or needed an emergency procedure, your life changed too. Heart disease is a reality for you and your family from now on. It will affect your sleeping, your eating, your travels, your activities, your children, your grandchildren, and your friends. Knowing the stages of coping will help you understand what you, your patient, and even your family feels. There is no set time to work through the process. Each person handles change differently. Some days you will even forget that life has changed. Other days you will feel overwhelmed and tired of worrying about your patient and the future. Knowing yourself and your patient better will help you be aware if you get "stuck" in one of the stages.

Time to Heal

Allow your patient to work through the healing process at his or her own speed, just as you should at your own pace. Realize that there will be times when you are in conflict with each other because you are at different stages. Just because you are feeling hopeful one week, your patient may be feeling angry that she has to take so much medication and has such a restricted diet. Your losses are real too. You may not have a bypass scar down your chest, but you have experienced loss. Trying to push the feelings of grief and loss away will only result in more intense feelings that explode when you least expect it or feelings that cause you to suffer physical consequences. Both you and your patient must take time to heal.

ELLEN'S STORY

"I tried to fly out the evening before my dad's bypass operation. I wanted to see him before he went to surgery. I wanted to be there for my mom. But my flight was canceled. I was forced to make reservations for the next morning and would not arrive in time to see my dad before surgery. As I stood in line at the ticket counter, I wanted to scream and cry.

The next morning, the man seated next to me on the plane asked if I was traveling on business or pleasure. As the tears started, I tried to explain about my father, who was already in surgery at that moment. My fear that something would happen to one of the strongest men I knew was overwhelming.

When I finally arrived at the hospital, the waiting room was crammed with family and friends. My mom was her usual self, totally in control, speaking to everyone, thanking them all for coming. However, when the word came that my dad was out of surgery and was okay, Mom sat down and began to cry. I realized then that she was facing extreme fear and anxiety."

Coping with Loss

Security and Stability

Before heart disease was diagnosed, you had the security that your spouse, partner, grandmother, son, or friend was going to be around the next day. You didn't worry when you went to sleep if he or she would live through the night. Now you listen to your loved one breathing during the night. You call him or her daily. Now you think about being alone. When we lose a sense of security, we temporarily feel less stable.

Patients deal with some of the same feelings. It is strange for them to wonder whether their heart is working and beating normally. It is strange for them to think about dying before you do. This unseen culprit called heart disease has invaded their entire sense of personal security and stability.

JIM'S STORY
(heart patient, 66)

"This heart stuff scares you. It's like you're a running back and have a knee blowout. You have surgery and it's supposed to be all better, but you won't plant your leg down quite as firmly again. You will always be a little tentative. It's like pushing a rope. You have to learn not to go at the pace you want to sometimes. I feel good. I don't feel fine, but I feel fortunate."

Routine

After the heart attack or surgery, normal routines are all in question for the patient and the caregiver. What you eat, when you eat, when you schedule doctors' appointments, how much you work, how much you lift, and how much you exercise are among the many questions patients and caregivers must ask on a regular basis. You will gradually find a new routine, but it will not be the same.

Identity

You are still the same person you were before your patient's heart surgery, but for a while and maybe for a long time, your roles may be reversed. You knew who you were. You were the spouse or son or daughter of someone strong and healthy. Now you know that no one is invincible and you are the friend, family member, and caregiver of a heart patient. Heart disease is part of your family's identity. Your patient is no longer identified simply by gender or family status or occupation. Now, he or she is also a heart disease patient.

Stages of Grief and Loss

The stages of grief and loss were made famous through the writings and appearances of the pioneer in hospice care, Dr. Elisabeth Kubler-Ross. Read them carefully and see where you and your patient are in working through the process.

Denial

Denial is the protective first stage of the grief process. Patients and caregivers deny the seriousness of the diagnosis by acting as if they are not affected. They may dilute the doctor's words with phrases like "He always bounces back" or "She's a strong woman, she can handle this." If it were not for initial denial, our fears would completely overtake us and immobilize us. Denial helps us cope until we can face the facts and adjust to the news.

Some patients and caregivers think that medication or surgery *cures* heart disease. Surgery and medicine are Band-Aids that help to stabilize the patient's condition but must be accompanied by a consistent healthy diet, regular exercise, and stress reduction to reverse the effects of heart disease.

Anger

After the initial shock wears off, both patients and caregivers move into the anger stage. Anger is a normal, healthy reaction to change and the loss of control over daily life. Caregivers may respond to their patients in anger or take their anger out on medical personnel or their extended family and friends. Fear, anxiety, and stress enhance feelings of anger. Sometimes all you need is for someone to listen to you. Find a friend you can "bitch and moan to" who can handle your complaints. Find a counselor who understands the grief process and can help you deal with your anger.

> *"Be patient with your patient!"*
>
> —75-YEAR-OLD CAREGIVER

DOROTHY'S STORY
(caregiver, 75)

"I am a very controlling person. I try not to be, but I always have been. I had been married to my husband for almost fifty years when he had a heart attack and bypass surgery. Everything happened so fast. I wasn't sure he was going to make it. When he came home after his surgery, I was like a commanding general. I wouldn't let anyone help him. I had to be in control of his meals, his getting up and down, and his walking. I was not all that nice about it either.

In looking back, I think I was angry and scared about the whole thing and the future. What happened was totally out of my control. I could not make him better. But I could make sure he got better. Finally, after two weeks, my daughter shook her finger in my face and told me to let my husband do more for himself. I started letting up and letting him do a little bit more every day."

Here are some suggestions for dealing with an angry patient:

♦ Listen to your patient. Allow him or her to vent some feelings. When people are in pain or even mild discomfort, they tend to be irritable.

♦ If your patient tends to take angry feelings out on you, calmly say that you want to help and listen, but not if you are going to be yelled at or hurt.

♦ Leave the room if you need to and come back when you have taken some deep breaths and can stay mentally in control of your emotions.

♦ Model how you want your patient to treat you. Model how he or she can work through the anger stage.

♦ Never tell your patient how he or she *should* feel. Even if you have had every heart procedure and problem known to the medical world, your patient will react and feel differently than you did.

♦ Remind your loved one that angry outbursts are dangerous and can lead to heart attacks. Work with your patient to find an alternative outlet for his or her feelings.

LYNN'S STORY

(caregiver, 41)

"I always got along with my father. We joke around a lot. But after his surgery he was emotional and depressed. He didn't joke for a long time. Not only were we dealing with him having heart disease, but we were dealing with a different man. I didn't know what to do or how to handle him. I finally called my uncle to come stay for a week and help. He got my dad to see how he was acting and how it made us feel. I think my dad listened to him because he was 'new' on the scene and because he was a man. He trusted my uncle."

Bargaining

Bargaining is an emotionally manipulative phase. It buys both the patient and the caregiver some more time to face the lifelong diagnosis of heart disease. In the bargaining stage, we make commitments and promises to ourselves, to each other, and often to God. Patients set goals to stop smoking, to exercise, or to treasure life every day. Caregivers make promises to give up bad habits, to go to church, and to love their patients more. Bargaining goals can give patients and caregivers a stronger sense of purpose and hope.

Goal setting is not wrong. However, we often tend to set ambitious goals that are hard to keep. After a few months, when we

HEART POINT

A study conducted by the Albert Einstein College of Medicine in the Bronx, New York, found that survivors of stroke, heart attacks, and cancer who became depressed were 60 percent more likely to suffer another stroke or heart attack or cancer progression than those who did not become depressed. They were 80 percent more likely to die.

start to falter on our commitments, patients may have a sense of failure and feel like doom is certain. Caregivers feel guilty that they have let their patients down. Some go too far and think that if they do not keep their bargaining goals that something bad can happen to their patients if they don't succeed. It's not unusual for caregivers to set tough goals, but be ready to hang in and keep trying.

Depression

Depression is common among heart patients. Many patients we interviewed or surveyed had experienced it in varying degrees after suffering a heart attack or undergoing bypass surgery. However, you will not find it addressed in many books about heart disease. Physicians are trained to spot medical problems, and conscientious caregivers strive to encourage their patients to eat right and exercise and de-stress more; but neither may be alert to the signs of depression in their patients. Depression attacks a person psychologically and makes a physically ill person feel and seem even sicker. It hinders the recovery process and creates stress. Because we tend to idolize the "tough guy" image in our society and treat depression like an emotional plague, many people suffering from it do not ask for help.

> "Never be afraid or embarrassed to seek help in dealing with your feelings and frustrations. Use your support systems. Use your medical team. Remember, if you want to be the best help to your patient, you must first help yourself."

Caregivers need to be aware of the signs of depression. Over a period of weeks, if you recognize some ongoing symptoms as those your patient is experiencing, talk to a professional. Start with your primary physician. If you don't feel that you receive adequate information and help, try a mental health professional such as a psychologist, psychiatrist, or social worker. A depressed person is not crazy or in a constant bad mood. They are in an emotional "funk" that can affect their physical health if left untreated.

Caregivers also need to be aware that they, too, can experience depression. Never be afraid or embarrassed to seek help in dealing with your feelings and frustrations. Use your support systems. Use your medical team. Remember, if you want to be the best help to your patient, you must first help yourself.

Get some needed rest. Do something with a friend. Schedule some weekly time just for you to get away without thinking about your patient or heart disease. Find a friend or professional you can talk to about what you are feeling physically and emotionally.

Earlier in this chapter, we encouraged patients to learn to listen to their bodies. We heartily advise caregivers to do the same. Stay aware of your emotional and physical health and changes.

ELAINE'S STORY

(caregiver, 58)

"Life has never been the same since we found out my husband has heart disease. I had no idea what we were in for. I tried to be optimistic, but I found myself worrying so much about him that I didn't take care of me."

Acceptance

Moving to the acceptance stage does not mean that the caregiver or the patient will not back-pedal at different times and revert to a former stage. A new medication, another medical procedure, the death of a friend in cardiac rehab, or any other trauma can set both of you back. Dealing with our own mortality and the mortality of those we care about is a lifelong process. Facing death is never easy. Acceptance has more to do with how you choose to live your life while coping with this lifelong illness. Acceptance brings an attitude of hopefulness that you can still live a full and meaningful life as a patient or as a caregiver. Yes, life will be different. Yes, things have changed. And yes, you have faced the possibility of death, but now you press forward to make the most of each day.

You will begin to think about what you want to do tomorrow, next week, next month, and even next year. When you are free to feel hope about the future, you will experience renewed emotional and physical energy.

JAMES'S STORY

(heart patient, 72)

"We are always concerned and rightfully so. But I know my condition better than anyone else. I have packed in enough living for two lives. I plan to
keep on making the most of every day."

Both a patient and a caregiver can easily make a list of the negative effects
of dealing with heart disease. We want to turn that around and help you look
at the positive. Positive thinking helps the body and mind feel stronger and
reduces stress.

SIGNS OF DEPRESSION

- Chronic sadness, anxiety, complaints of feeling "empty"
- Tiredness, lack of energy
- Loss of interest in or pleasure in ordinary activities
- Difficulty falling asleep or getting back to sleep, or the opposite—
  excessive sleeping
- Loss of appetite or overeating
- Frequent crying
- Unexplained, constant aches and pains
- Difficulty concentrating, paying attention, remembering, or making
  decisions
- Increased irritability
- Disinterest in regular grooming and hygiene
- Expressions of guilt, hopelessness, and worthlessness
- Uncharacteristic withdrawal from other people
- Sudden manic-like behavior
- Increased alcohol or drug use (including prescription drugs)
- Thoughts of suicide or a suicide attempt

CAREGIVER EVALUATION

1. As a caregiver, I take time for myself.
    A. Working hard at it
    B. Try to as much as I can
    C. Realize I need to
    D. Can't do it yet

2. I can identify the grief process stages I have been through and where I am now in the process of coping with loss and change.
    A. Working hard at it
    B. Trying to understand my feelings
    C. Realize I need to
    D. Can't do it yet

3. I can identify the grief process stage my patient is in and how he or she is coping with loss and change.
    A. Working hard at it
    B. Trying to understand his feelings
    C. Realize I need to
    D. Can't do it yet

4. I am finding practical ways to reduce the stress in my life.
    A. Working hard at it
    B. Try to as much as I can
    C. Realize I need to
    D. Can't do it yet

5. I understand that it takes time for me to heal emotionally.
    A. Working hard at it
    B. Trying to
    C. Realize I need to
    D. Can't do it yet

SHARE IMPORTANT INFORMATION

PATIENTS AND CAREGIVERS need to discuss financial matters, wills, and legal issues. Patients can create a file or make and post lists of important documents and their location. Make another list of who should be called in case of emergency or death. Caregivers should know the names and phone numbers of their patient's doctors, attorney, minister, accountant, insurance agent, bank, and executor of the will.

The patient needs to share a list of any safe deposit boxes, bank box numbers, and who is authorized to open the boxes. Caregivers need to be kept up to date on the patient's insurance policies, including health and life.

In addition, be sure a caregiver knows where to find the patient's birth certificate, automobile registration, deed to a home, Social Security number, and driver's license.

A Living Will

Everyone should have a living will. It is even more important for anyone facing a significant health crisis. A living will is a legal document that specifies your wishes about medical care if you are no longer able to make them known. It can limit the type and amount of medical care you want to receive if you are incapacitated or terminal. It may limit the use of life-sustaining equipment, such as automatic ventilators. It could also specify a "do not resuscitate order," though most hospitals ask patients to provide this on their forms. You should discuss the living will with your family and with your regular doctors. They should have a clear understanding of your wishes. They should have a copy of this document in their files in case you go to the hospital, are unconscious, and have no family member with you.

Although it might feel strange or morbid, it will reduce stress if the patient has updated a living will and feels secure in the designated amounts of life insurance and health insurance. Getting things in order and keeping them in order will provide everyday help and will be especially supportive when you are facing a critical situation.

Other Legal Issues

How does the caregiver's relationship with the patient affect legal considerations? If you are married, then there is probably no issue, but if the patient is a parent or other relative, or unrelated, consider whether there are legal considerations in your caring for your patient's affairs. Check with an attorney to see what legal rights you have at the hospital and with making financial decisions if you are an unmarried domestic partner or friend of the patient.

General Power of Attorney
A general power of attorney is a document that one person authorizes allowing another person to act on his or her behalf. A special power of attorney is a document that one person authorizes allowing another person to act on his or her behalf in special situations. The person who accepts the duties that come with having power of attorney need not be a lawyer. Patients can sign a document appointing an individual to make health care decisions if the patient should become incapacitated or incompetent. The person named in the health care power of attorney should be the caregiver or some other adult the patient trusts. In some states, when you enter the hospital you will be given a Health Care Proxy form to complete. If you choose to complete the form and sign it, it authorizes another person to make health care decisions for when you are unable to make them. You can grant authority as complete or as limited as you decide.

Financial Matters

It is helpful for the patient to determine his net worth to see if he is eligible for any federal or state programs. If the patient is not sure about her net worth, caregivers can help. List all the patient's assets, including cash, bonds, CDs, IRAs, investments, stocks, life insurance cash value, real estate, and personal property such as furniture, jewelry, and cars. Determine an approximate dollar value for each and add them up. List all the patient's liabilities, including taxes due, monthly bills, credit card debt, remaining balance owed on a mortgage, remaining balance owed on a car, and any other outstanding loans. Take the sum of the liabilities and subtract it from the sum of the assets to determine the patient's overall financial situation.

Patient and caregiver need to think of extra costs that could accumulate due to help needed after surgery or any uninsured costs such as medication or home health care. Check with social service agencies, a hospital social worker, or a financial planner to help find ways to cover uninsured costs. If the patient is over sixty-five, find out what help is available from Medicaid, Medicare, Social Security, and state and local programs. The American Association of Retired Persons (AARP) has an extensive website (listed in Resources) and printed materials addressing the financial needs and current health care of seniors.

KNOW YOUR PATIENT

MUCH OF THE time, a patient's behavior is predictable. If a person usually complains and whines when ill, that person will not change with all the pains and procedures accompanying heart disease. But the seriousness of the disease can motivate a person to find new determination. A caregiver must prepare for different reactions, discover ways to cope with the patient's responses, and learn methods to lessen the severity of a negative response. Observing how the patient communicates and responds to the medical team and visitors in the hospital gives the caregiver additional information.

Try on Your Patient's Shoes

Take time as your patient is recuperating and think about how you would feel if you were the patient. Finding out you have a disease that affects you for the rest of your life is a startling reality. Going through a heart emergency when it is *your heart* is not something anyone would choose to do. Would you feel fear? Anger? Depression? Hopelessness?

Think about your patient and how she usually responds to life.

Understanding why the patient is feeling a certain way will help you deal with a variety of her feelings. Remember that patients must go through the grief process just as caregivers go through it.

Be prepared for your patient to express anger. Patients can become very demanding and lash out at caregivers, friends, and family. Your patient will feel many emotions, but dealing with his or her anger will be one of the most challenging for you because it hurts the most.

STAR POINT TWO

Educate Yourself

> *"The beginning of understanding is calling things by their correct name."*
>
> —OLD CHINESE SAYING

KNOWLEDGE AND UNDERSTANDING are powerful. In Star Point Two, we lay the foundation for understanding coronary artery and heart disease. We describe how it feels, what it does to the patient, and tools doctors use to diagnose it. As you read about the heart and circulatory system, you will learn to call things by their correct names. This will enable you to effectively communicate with medical personnel, help you understand what is happening to your body, and most important of all, to take charge of your own heart care. Assertive, educated patients and those who feel in control have much better outcomes.

DARRELL'S STORY

"I am naturally curious, and once I get the desire to learn about something, I tend to dig deeply. This trait made it easy for me to learn about my heart, heart disease, and what was happening to me. Later, I learned that knowledge was power. It enabled me to discuss my problems and challenges with all of my doctors. It gave me confidence to challenge, question more deeply, and, finally, take charge of my own health. This has earned the respect and cooperation of my doctors and has helped me to survive."

"Men stumble over the truth from time to time, but most pick themselves up and hurry off as if nothing happened."
—WINSTON CHURCHILL (1874–1965)

HEART GEOGRAPHY

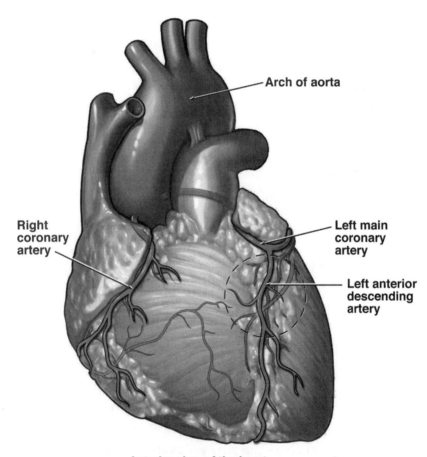

Right coronary artery

Arch of aorta

Left main coronary artery

Left anterior descending artery

Anterior view of the heart

A front view of the heart and the coronary arteries. Copyright © 2002 Nucleus Communications, Inc. All rights reserved. www.nucleusinc.com

THE HEART IS an amazing pumping machine that beats over 100,000 times a day and 2.5 billion times in your lifetime. This small but significant muscle weighs only 7 to 15 ounces and is slightly larger than the size of a fist. The heart and circulatory system make up a complex network that most people don't understand, even after treatment or surgery. The heart is a muscle that powers the movement of blood through our body. Its action is much like a squeeze bottle that is compressed to pump the blood from our heart into all parts of our body. The blood then flows back into the heart (refilling the squeeze bottle) in preparation for another squeeze or contraction of the heart. Valves control the flow of blood so blood can only move in one direction, either pumped out or flowing back in.

Much of the rest of the system is plumbing, pipes, and connectors. Sometimes the pieces fail and need repair or the pipes become clogged. The key is taking charge and avoiding the need for repair.

HEART POINT

The ancients thought the heart was the center of our existence. Aristotle maintained a cardiocentric theory of life: the heart was the ruler of the body and soul. Plato and Hippocrates argued that the brain was the center of all intellectual faculties and the center of life. Shakespeare joined the controversy years later when he wrote in the *Merchant of Venice* (act 3, scene 2), "Tell me where is fancy bred, Or in the heart or in the head?"

HOW THE HEART WORKS

The Muscle

The squeeze bottle is actually quite marvelous and complex. The heart is really two distinct sections, the right and left side, divided by an impermeable wall. There are four hollow areas or chambers, two on each side of the heart. Each side has a thin-walled atrium, a left atrium and a right atrium. The atria act as storage tanks for blood returning to the heart. The heavy-walled, left and right ventricles do the heavy pumping work of the heart.

Blood Flow

The beating of the heart regulates the ebb and flow of blood throughout the body.Blue, oxygen-spent blood returns from the extremities to the right atrium via the body's two major veins, the inferior and superior venae cavae. Bright red, oxygenated blood moves from the lungs, via the pulmonary veins, to the left atrium. This first phase of the heartbeat sequence, when the heart fills with blood, is the diastole. The diastolic is the blood pressure that remains in your arteries when your heart is between beats—the lower number. Blood flows from the atria, in the upper chambers of the heart, into the ventricles in the lower chambers of the heart. Tissue-paper-thin valves regulate that flow. The ventricles fill to about 80 percent of capacity by the end of the diastole phase.

During the next phase, the atrial systole, the atria squeeze the remaining blood into the ventricles. This is initiated by an electrical impulse from our "natural pacemaker," the sinoatrial node.

As that phase ends, the third phase, the ventricular systole, begins with another electrical impulse. Systolic blood pressure (the higher number) is the reading of the pressure when the heart contracts and forces blood into the aorta. The electrical impulse causes the ventricles to contract. Valves close between the ventricles and atria, and the ventricle exit valves open. The contracting ventricles force blood out and into the aorta and pulmonary artery. As the ventricular systole ends, the diastole phase begins anew. This cycle continues as long as the heart does.

Where the Blood Goes

The heart continually pumps blood to fill the need of various organs of the body. As the body works harder, for instance with exercise, the nervous system sends signals to increase the speed at which the heart works. Each organ has specific needs. With the body at rest, the brain needs about ½ pint of blood, the skin 1 pint, the muscles 2 pints, and the coronary arteries ½ pint (all, blood flow per minute). During exercise the needs change—except for the brain, which still needs ½ pint of blood—the skin now needs 4 pints, the muscles 24 pints, and the coronary arteries 1½ pints.

The Coronary System

The heart is the hardest-working muscle in the body. It needs its own supply of oxygen-rich blood to sustain its activities. All of the blood that passes through the heart cannot be used by it. The heart has a unique plumbing system of its own arteries, veins, and capillaries. These are specially adapted for the critical purpose of supplying oxygen to all areas of the heart.

The left and right coronary arteries connect at the beginning of the aorta. Small arteries branch off from them and into the heart. The left artery immediately divides into two large arteries, the left anterior descending and the circumflex artery.

The Vascular System

Our blood supply cycles through our bodies about once every minute, 1,440 times per day, covering a distance of 60,000 miles with each loop. The left ventricle squeezes blood out of the heart and into the aorta about seventy times a minute, over 2.5 billion times in an average lifetime. Our blood vessels are adapted to stand up to that pressure and pounding. Would the metal pipes in our homes stand that physical onslaught? Probably not.

Arteries and veins carry all of the blood pumped by the heart away and back to the heart respectively. Each artery has an unusual four-layer construction: a fibrous outer coating, a strong muscle, a tough layer of elastic tissue, and a membranous, smooth inner lining. This unique structure is strong, yet flexible. The larger arteries, including the aorta, act like a support pump, helping to move the blood through our bodies at about one foot per second. The arteries branch and get smaller as they move away from the heart. As they get smaller, the proportion of muscle increases until one muscle cell wraps around the tiniest artery, an arteriole. Those tiny muscles

---

HEART POINT

The heart beats about fifty to seventy times a minute at rest.

squeeze blood into our 10 billion capillaries. Our bodies are so dense with capillaries that any of our individual cells are less than a millionth of an inch from a blood supply. A network of capillaries is the connector of arteries to veins, allowing oxygen-depleted blood to begin its return trip to the heart.

WHAT CAN GO WRONG?

WITH THE INTRICACY of the heart and circulatory system, any "small" problem can become a life-threatening crisis. What follows is a discussion of some of the things that can go wrong. We also look at various approaches to diagnosing the problem.

HEART POINT

Five hundred red blood cells stacked on top of one another would measure only .04 inch high.

Hardening of the Arteries (Atherosclerosis)

"The beginning of health is to know the disease."
—MIGUEL DE CERVANTES (1547–1616)

Atherosclerosis and its aftermath are the main focus of this book. In healthy individuals, the arteries are smooth and elastic, allowing the blood to flow easily. The flexibility helps the artery handle changes in pressure. If you have high cholesterol, a large amount of fatty material, bundled with other substances, flows through your bloodstream. This material adheres to damaged spots on the artery wall or where they branch. Some of these damaged areas occur naturally as our arteries twist and turn from the force of blood that is propelled through them each time our heart beats. Poor lifestyle choices will increase damages to your

HEART POINT

There are 60,000 miles of veins and arteries in our bodies.

arteries. Carbon monoxide, a byproduct of smoking, hormones from stress, and high blood pressure damage the linings of our arteries. Damage does not have to happen. Sensible lifestyle choices and medical intervention can decrease or control these risks.

As the fatty deposits get larger, they increase the damage to the artery wall. These masses continue to increase in size, harden to plaque, reduce the flexibility of the wall, and finally restrict blood flow. *As these blockages grow, so does your risk of a stroke or heart attack.*

Atherosclerosis is primarily a lifestyle disease. It is rampant in countries that have a rich, cholesterol-laden diet, relying mostly on high-fat foods like meat, butter, and eggs. Dr. William P. Castelli, the former medical director of the Framingham Heart Study, suggested that an improvement in diet alone would decrease risk for most heart attack patients.

HEART POINT

Plaque is a hardened mass of fatty tissue that attaches to the lining of artery walls.

Coronary Artery Disease (Also Called Coronary Heart Disease)

Atherosclerosis in the coronary arteries is particularly dangerous. The coronary arteries supply the oxygenated blood to the heart. This keeps the heart healthy and pumping. When a blockage or clot chokes off that blood supply, you can have a heart attack.

Angina

Angina, or angina pectoris, is a symptom of a substantial problem, not a disease itself. It is chest pain, and sometimes other pain or symptoms (see the section on symptoms in Star Point One), caused by inadequate blood flow and oxygen to the heart muscle, caused by partially or totally blocked artery or arteries. As angina is a symptom of a problem—usually atherosclerosis, though sometimes aortic stenosis, hyperthyroidism, high blood pressure, or anemia—a physician must examine you to determine its cause.

Heart Attack (Myocardial Infarction)

A heart attack occurs when the heart does not get an adequate supply of blood. A permanent blockage or one lasting more than thirty minutes to two hours, in the coronary arteries, causes the attack. Heart muscle tissue starved for oxygen dies. An infarct is the permanently damaged area.

Stroke

A stroke occurs when the brain does not get an adequate supply of blood. In essence, it is a brain attack instead of a heart attack. It is related to atherosclerosis. One form of stroke is caused by blockages in the carotid or cerebral artery, the neck and brain arteries. Other strokes are caused by a clot breaking off and lodging near the brain, blocking blood flow. Other types are provoked by hemorrhages.

Stroke symptoms vary by type but may include weakness or paralysis of arms or legs, numbness, and speech, vision, and comprehension problems.

High Blood Pressure

You have high blood pressure when your heart pumps blood through your circulatory system with more force than required. That exaggerated pumping action requires more energy and places more strain on the entire circulatory system than normal. Each of the 100,000 heartbeats per day puts additional strain on your arteries as they twist and turn with more than usual force. That force will increase the number of small injuries on the walls of the arteries, which provide more locations for fatty deposits and plaque to accumulate.

High blood pressure, the "silent killer," is usually symptomless. Most people have no warnings (though a few people have more nosebleeds than normal or awaken with a slight ache in the back of the head). In examining data from the Framingham Heart Study, even slightly elevated blood pressure, so-called high normal with systolic readings of 130 to 139 or diastolic from 85 to 89, lead to higher risks of cardiac disease.

Valve Problems

Our hearts have four valves. Two separate the upper chambers of the heart (the atria) from the lower chambers of the heart (the ventricles); one on the right side and one on the left. Two control the flow from the ventricles into the major arteries, the pulmonary artery from the right side, and the aorta from the left side. Each of these valves controls the flow of blood so that it will move in only one direction.

The two major valve problems are not opening properly, called stenosis, and not closing properly. A congenital heart defect sometimes causes stenosis, though frequently the problem is calcification or thickening of the valve with age. When valves don't close properly, blood can flow backward, a process called regurgitation. Coronary heart disease, rheumatic heart disease, or bacterial endocarditis can cause this. The valves on the left side of the heart, those that control the powerful surges of blood produced by the powerful left ventricle, have the most problems.

Arrhythmias—Electrical Problems

Our regular heartbeat speeds up during exercise or in stressful situations. If you have done the self-monitoring exercises in Star Point One, you understand your heartbeat at rest and the changes during exercise. You also will be better able to identify unusual or irregular beating patterns. An arrhythmia is when your heart beats at an unusually fast or slow pace.

Coronary artery disease is the most common cause of potentially life-threatening arrhythmias (ventricular tachycardia and ventricular fibrillation). Plaque narrows these essential arteries, blocking the flow of blood. The lack of blood damages the special cells that control the electrical pulses that guide the action of the heart. This can happen over time or suddenly after a heart attack. Once those cells are damaged, cocaine (always dangerous) or even small irri-tations, such as those from coffee (caffeine), alcohol, or smoking, can provoke an arrhythmia.

Heart Failure

In heart failure, the heart's pumping action cannot take care of pumping blood to your body. A valve problem may have put extra stress on the heart muscle or it could have been damaged by disease. Heart failure does not mean that the heart stops pumping altogether and that the condition is immediately life-threatening but that the heart is less effective than before. The seriousness of the underlying disorder and its treatment will determine the outcome of treating this disorder.

Coronary artery disease and high blood pressure are the two major problems that cause heart failure. Coronary artery disease slows the blood flow going to the heart. High blood pressure puts extra strain on the heart. Other causes include diabetes, anemia, valve problems, lung disease, pericarditis, vitamin B_1 deficiency, or direct heart muscle damage from alcohol or drugs.

Heart failure may affect only one side of the heart but usually affects both. Congestive heart failure involves the entire heart.

DARRELL'S STORY

"I finally was referred to a cardiologist to rule out any heart problem from my 'back pain.' The nurse prepared me for the treadmill stress test and hooked me up to the equipment. The cardiologist came in, introduced himself, and asked, 'Why are you here?' I thoroughly described my symptoms, what my primary care doctor had called 'back pain.' He paused, and then looked at me, and I thought, 'Damn! I knew I was in trouble and that he really meant business.' He said, 'I'm not giving you the stress test. I want you to go to Mt. Sinai Hospital for an angiogram.' I immediately knew I had to go. I knew how serious it was by looking at his face. (I also knew that I would love to play poker with him—he could never bluff!) Several days later, the angiogram showed that my left anterior descending artery was 100 percent closed."

HEART POINT

The stethoscope was invented in 1816 by Dr. Rene T. H. Laënnec, considered the father of chest medicine, to avoid getting fleas from his patients. The standard practice was for a doctor to listen to the patient's heart by placing an ear on the chest to listen. This also was embarrassing for female patients.

TESTING FOR HEART DISEASE

THE INVESTIGATION OF symptoms that lead to a diagnosis of heart disease often proceeds through a series of simple to more serious or invasive tests. Doctors select the least invasive or difficult test that the situation dictates. Today's doctors have an incredible range of tests and procedures that were not available even thirty years ago. We hope that more new techniques will be developed in the future to make the entire diagnostic process easier and more accurate. And even with today's technology, a doctor's knowledge, experience, and skill play a significant role in the results and recommendations—the selection of a doctor is just as important as it always was. (See Star Point Three for information on selecting a doctor and hospital.) Following are some of the diagnostic procedures—roughly in order of the simplest to the more difficult, expensive, and invasive—that patients need to understand.

Listening to the Heart and Patient

One of the first things most doctors do is talk to the patient. If you are a new patient, possibly referred to a cardiologist for the first time, she will review your health history. She will read the form you (usually) filled out at the office along with the family health history that you brought with you (see Star Point One.)

Then she will elicit responses from you concerning changes in your body or health, pain, or other symptoms. The more you are in touch with your body and the problems you are having, the easier it will be for you to describe your difficulties and symptoms to the doctor.

The doctor may put a hand on your chest and feel your heart. This could tell him if the heart, or some section of the heart, is enlarged.

Another procedure will be listening to your heart. We have all had a doctor place the often cold, metal piece of a stethoscope on our chest. That metal piece contains a diaphragm, a sound-amplifying device. It is connected to a piece of tubing that splits into a Y, the top pieces leading to ear pieces on each side of the doctor's head.

The doctor listens carefully to all of the sounds of your heart. Healthy heart sounds can vary by age but generally include the "lubb" and "dupp" sounds of valves closing. If he hears "clicks" and "snaps," he will investigate further. These can indicate valve problems. If he hears a "whooshing" noise, you have a heart murmur. Murmurs are more common for babies or young people and often require no treatment and soon disappear. There are several causes of murmurs, including an abnormally tight or a leaky valve. If the murmur persists or you have other symptoms, the doctor will run additional tests.

Electrocardiogram (EKG)

The electrocardiogram (EKG or ECG) is a widely used cardiac test. Most people have seen one administered on television or experienced it themselves. Usually, the doctor places ten or twelve suction-cup devices, attached to lead wires, on the chest, ankles, and wrists. Leads run to the electrocardiograph machine, which measures the minute amounts of electrical energy generated by heart muscles as they work. There is no danger of electrical shock because the electrical energy is flowing from your heart to the machine. No electricity flows from the EKG machine to the patient. The resulting printout, the electrocardiogram, provides a picture of the electrical activity of the heart from several viewpoints.

A healthy heart produces a typical or predictable pattern. The EKG is good at pinpointing electrical problems of the heart (e.g., unusual heart rhythms, electrical conduction problems, and the malfunctioning of an implanted pacemaker). It also can help pinpoint thickening of heart muscles and damage from coronary artery disease or a heart attack. The EKG cannot show previous angina pain. If you have angina pain while taking the test, the test will sometimes show it, though not consistently.

Holter Monitor

You generally lie down briefly for a standard EKG. If the cardiologist suspects intermittent heart abnormalities, he may ask you to "wear" a Holter monitor for a full day or longer. This portable device measures the same electrical activity as the EKG over a period of hours or days and shows problems caused by specific activities or stresses.

Telemetry EKG

This test involves the use of a device that sends your EKG via radio-type waves to a base receiver-printer. A nurse or doctor continuously monitors you while you exercise, jog, or complete simulated tasks. Cardiac rehabilitation centers use this to closely observe patients as they exercise. The range of the device is usually about 330 unobstructed feet.

ELLEN'S STORY

"My dad was already attending a cardiac rehab program due to an arrhythmia problem followed by congestive heart failure. As is the practice in the program, patients are hooked up to an EKG monitor while they are exercising. One morning, the program doctor checked my dad's EKG strip and was quite concerned. He sent it immediately on to a cardiologist, and within a week, my father had quadruple bypass surgery. The cardiologist told him that he was the type person who would have had very few warning signs of a heart attack and would have probably just dropped dead. Careful monitoring in the rehab program can save lives."

Exercise EKG (Stress Test)

The exercise EKG (exercise stress test or simply stress test) continually measures your electrical heart activity while exercising. Most often, this is done on a treadmill or occasionally on an exercise bicycle. A technician attaches EKG leads to your body. The test starts at a slow speed, at a walking pace on flat ground on the treadmill. Every few minutes the doctor increases the speed and incline, progressing from an easy walk to a demanding, uphill jog. This continues until the patient must stop because of breathlessness or leg fatigue. The test may run from nine to fifteen minutes or be stopped because of angina pain or other problems.

Another form of the test starts with the patient already warmed up. The treadmill speed is set at a higher, yet comfortable level for the patient. This speed is constant throughout the test with the incline increasing.

These tests are useful in detecting blockages because they may indicate an abnormal EKG reading. Blockages can be present without the patient having angina pain. No test is perfect, including this one, where a patient with blockages may have normal EKG readings during the test. Sometimes small vessels, collaterals, have developed to compensate for the blockages. Women at menopause, heart patients taking digitalis, and others may have false test results that inaccurately suggest a problem.

If you have a family history of premature heart disease and any of the risk factors for atherosclerosis, a doctor may want you to take a stress test at an early age.

JOHAN'S STORY
(heart patient, 55)

"I visited my family doctor two weeks after my brother died from his heart attack.

My mother had also died from a heart attack. I explained my family history. He gave me an EKG and said I was fine. I continued to press him to do a treadmill stress test. He said, 'No, you are fine.' Two years later I had a major heart attack. My cardiologist was appalled that my doctor didn't give me the stress test."

Radionuclide Scanning

In these tests, a small amount of radioactive material, called radioisotopes, is injected into your vein. Your bloodstream moves it to the heart. Sensitive gamma cameras show views of the heart that are "built" using the variations in absorption of the material. The three variations of these tests are thallium scanning, technetium scanning, and cardiac blood pool imaging. Though similar in basic principles, each test provides slightly different information.

Thallium Scanning

The most common of the tests is the thallium scan, which is usually done as part of a stress test. Near the end of the treadmill stress test, the cardiologist injects thallium into your vein. When you finish the treadmill portion, you move to a camera room. A technician takes a number of views of your heart and arteries. Generally, the technician repeats the process in about four hours or the next day.

Healthy heart muscle absorbs the material; damaged muscle does not. These variations help the doctor define the damage level from a heart attack or assess the success of coronary artery bypass surgery. The results can also show blocked areas of coronary arteries.

DARRELL'S STORY

"I have had three thallium stress tests with varying results. The first one was about a month after my first angioplasty. I was feeling wonderfully, thinking I had totally beaten my problem. Though I had not really changed my diet, I was exercising more than ever. The test results showed a blockage. Because I was doing so well and feeling so great, the test seemed to be a false positive. A few weeks later during a celebration vacation in Key West, Florida, I had my first clue that something was not right. Most days, I was walking four miles at aerobic speed in tropical heat and humidity. I was a little more tired than normal but chalked it up to the conditions. The major clue occurred when I was attempting to snorkel the reef; I simply ran out of energy and had to get back on the boat. A few weeks later I had angina pain. Shortly after that, I had another angioplasty to open the blockage in the stent placed during the first one.

I had the second thallium stress test after my second angioplasty. The results showed that I didn't have any significant blockages. Again, I thought I was out of the woods. Several weeks later angina pain started again. Blockages can form quickly. I learned that I am always going to be in a battle with coronary heart disease.

A third test about two years after my triple bypass did not show any major problems. More than one year after that, I still have no angina pain."

Technetium Scanning

The other significant nuclear scanning technique uses the isotope technetium. The damaged heart muscle, not healthy muscle, absorbs the radioactive material. This type of scanning can confirm a recent heart attack or the extent of the damage.

Cardiac Blood Pool Imaging (MUGA Scan)

Another form of technetium attaches to the red blood cells. The camera then captures images, a multiple-gated acquisition (MUGA) scan, of blood flowing in and out of the heart and the pools of blood at different stages of the heartbeat. Doctors can see how well the ventricle is pumping blood and the movements of the walls of the heart.

Positron Emission Tomography (PET) Scanning

A PET scan starts with the injection of a radioactive tracing substance into the patient's vein. The tracing substance travels to the heart and is absorbed proportionately by muscles relative to their activity level. The ring-shaped PET scanner "reads" the variation in muscle activity. The machine produces images that help show the heart's level of metabolism and blood flow.

Magnetic Resonance Imaging (MRI)

The MRI is now being used more widely for evaluation of a broad range of problems, including coronary artery disease. You lie inside a large magnet, which manipulates the nuclei of the atoms of your body so that a computer can create images of your body. This is a painless test and uses no radioactive material. The test shows the amount of plaque formed on artery walls from atherosclerosis. This may be helpful in the early identification of at-risk patients who have shown no other symptoms of atherosclerosis.

Echocardiography

In echocardiography, a technician uses ultrasound to produce an image of the heart. This noninvasive test shows the opening and closing of valves, the heart chambers' size and shape, valves, and movement of the heart chambers. It can help evaluate the heart after a heart attack, reveal congenital heart defects, or show fluid around the heart or blood clots.

Cardiac Catheterization (Angiogram)

An angiogram is an invasive X-ray exam. The doctor threads a tiny catheter into your body and introduces a contrast medium into the coronary arteries, then takes an X-ray in order to study the flow of blood into the heart. This helps the doctor decide on additional treatments. It is not painful even though the patient is awake during the process.

DARRELL'S STORY

"I didn't find out that you can actually reverse heart disease by making significant lifestyle changes until after my second angioplasty. Many people believe that surgery and drugs cure them; that is simply not true. It is important that you work hard to improve your lifestyle, which improves your odds of controlling your heart disease."

STAR POINT THREE

Lead Your Team

"The first and best victory is to conquer self. To be conquered by self is, of all things, the most shameful and vile."

—PLATO (C. 428 B.C.–347 B.C.)

RESEARCH SHOWS THAT assertive patients have much better survival rates. You need to lead your health care team or, at least, "partner" with your doctors to achieve the best result. In an emergency or after surgery, caregivers must be prepared to step in and lead the team and to support the patient through further medical procedures and lifestyle changes. In Star Point Three we show each of you how to lead your respective teams and work together for the best results.

DARRELL'S STORY

"There are moments, or points, in our lives that are significant. In my case, they occurred each time that I chose to take charge. One of those moments happened several months into my struggle with heart disease, though I did not know that that was the battle I was fighting. I knew that for months I had 'back pain.' My initial worry about heart problems seemed misguided because of my doctor's diagnosis. That wasn't the issue—the issue was my lifestyle. My life was not normal anymore because of pain. My 'back pain' was debilitating and not getting better. I could not exercise, I could not walk to the subway, or up the stairs in the college where I was teaching—my life was being disrupted and I had to do something. I had to resolve my problem and decided to push my doctor hard to move the process along. I was not going to wait any longer.

"I made the appointment determined to move the process along; to demand the MRI of my back to settle this. The doctor decided I should have a treadmill stress test first. I sat there thinking, 'If I needed a cardiologist and a stress test all along, it's amazing that I'm not dead already.'

"The second moment came when I realized how badly my doctor had bungled my case. I really could have died. I had heart problems, and he almost did me in. I decided that I would fire him, yes, fire him. I was now in charge.

"From there, the steps came naturally and I simply had to educate myself so that I could be intelligently assertive. Monitoring my condition and body, choosing a hospital and surgeon followed naturally. The next section will help you take charge early and avoid my missteps."

FIND A DOCTOR YOU CAN TRUST

WE OFTEN PUT faith in doctors without checking them out. Most people spend more time selecting a new car or even a bottle of wine than in selecting a doctor. That latter choice can literally mean the difference between life and death. If you have a minor illness, you will probably get better naturally, so the choice of doctor is not critical. For several years, Darrell had been satisfied with the doctor who badly misdiagnosed his angina, but when you have a life-threatening illness these choices become more important. Recent reports in the news describe surgery on the wrong leg, organ, or even the wrong side of the brain. The comedian Dana Carvey sued his heart surgeon, who didn't operate on all of his closed arteries during his coronary bypass. This section of *Surviving with Heart* looks at some of the ways to choose doctors and surgeons, and how to select a hospital. Issues include the doctor's background and education, board certifications, reputation, examination and communication skills, prescribing philosophy, approach to preventative medicine, patient involvement in decision making, hospital appointments, and technical skills.

Choosing a Primary Care Physician

Even in an era of specialized medicine most of us need a doctor who can look at our whole body and deal with a variety of medical ailments. A good choice would be a primary care internist who looks at the complete person. Another generalist to look for might be a "family practitioner" or someone who "specializes in family medicine." Years ago we would call this type of doctor a G.P., or general practitioner. This generalist can help you navigate the maze of specialists and add knowledgeable insight to the tricky decision making that your life depends on.

DARRELL'S STORY

"After I fired my primary care doctor, I chose an endocrinologist for my primary care. They specialize in hormone and gland disorders. Some doctors specifically focus on diabetes (a diabetologist). I believe he was best trained to coordinate my general care while paying particular attention to my underlying risk factors for heart disease: diabetes, high blood pressure, and low HDL."

Doctor's Background and Education

How important is it that your doctor graduated from a prestigious university rather than a foreign medical school? It is widely agreed that if a doctor graduated from one of the top U.S. medical schools—such as Harvard, Yale, Johns Hopkins, or Columbia—he received a high-quality education. If you asked those working in medicine what countries have the best medical schools, the consensus would put the United States and Canada at the top of the list, with England close behind. If you want to consider a doctor trained in another country, focus on additional training and credentials. Many excellent physicians are trained in schools in other countries. Look at where they completed their residency requirements and if they are on the staff of a top hospital. Determine the areas in which they have board-certified specialties. These require specific additional training.

Locating Background Information

Several sources have basic background information on doctors, including their medical school education, residency, specialties, years in practice, other credentials, and office hours. Most insurance companies have background on the doctors in their networks. You can also call the doctor's office and ask the staff for that information. Hospitals have referral systems for doctors on staff or those with privileges. So, if you have a wonderful local hospital, ask there for a referral. They can also provide background information on the doctor. The American Medical Association's website, www.ama-assn.org, has a searchable database of more than 690,000 physicians. The research librarian at your local public library can help you locate the most up-to-date information on local doctors.

> *"Some doctors should have a warning sticker on their forehead saying, 'Warning, dangerous to your health.'"*
> —DARRELL TROUT

Many people rely on friends and family to recommend a doctor. Studies suggest that they evaluate a doctor by how nice they are or other interpersonal factors rather than skill level. Others rely on referrals from other physicians. Keep in mind that these referrals are frequently based on reciprocal agreements; both doctors referring patients to each other. Perhaps the best source is "medical insiders": residents, hospital nurses, or other nurses. They may talk to you "off the record" and tell you whom they would go to or send their family to.

It is difficult, though not impossible, to identify problem doctors. Your state medical licensing agency or board can tell you if there are actions taken against any doctor in the state. Many states are now posting the information on their websites. You should ask the doctor if she has practiced in any other state and check with those boards. Check with the local hospital where the doctor has privileges to see if any actions have been taken against her or if sanctions have been applied. In addition, ask the same questions directly of the doctor. She shouldn't have any trouble answering. If she hesitates to answer or seems to hedge a lot, it may be a sign of trouble. In 2000, the Public Citizen Health Research Group produced a CD-ROM, *20,125 Questionable Doctors Disciplined by State and Federal Governments.* It lists all doctors disciplined between 1991 and 2000. Check to see if it is available in a local library (cost at press time about $600).

Philosophy of Practice

Even knowing a doctor's credentials, you won't know his demeanor, "bedside manner," or philosophy. It may take a few visits to a particular doctor to start getting a feel for his approach to medicine and patients. Questions to consider:

- ◆ How does she relate to you as a person (both patient and caregiver)?
- ◆ Does she take your feelings into account?
- ◆ Will she work with you to get the most out of your insurance coverage?
- ◆ How does she feel about complementary approaches to medicine?
- ◆ Does she take the time to explain things to you?
- ◆ Is her philosophy of preventative medicine compatible with your own?

Doctors will also treat you differently if you are assertive and come prepared. Remember, you are the consumer and make the ultimate decision. If you can't work with a doctor or he is unresponsive to your needs, move on. Even within networks there is more than one doctor to choose from.

Other Considerations

There are many other things to consider when choosing a doctor. Is the doctor in your insurance network? How close is he to your home? What hospital is he affiliated with? What are the office hours? Can he be reached by telephone? Is the office staff helpful and pleasant or a detriment? Our experience with office staff varies dramatically. Some are rude and do much to get in the way between you and the doctor. On the other hand, Darrell's cardiologist's nurse and office manager, Kim, was invaluable as she helped him work through the maze of hospital bureaucracies and insurance. If you find nice and helpful staff, remember to thank them. Darrell took Kim flowers to say "thank you" for all her help.

MAKE THE MOST OF AN OFFICE VISIT

DOCTORS ARE UNDER increasing time pressure and spend less time with each patient than ever before. Research shows that doctors focus completely on a patient only during the first twenty-three seconds of an office visit. In this time-pressed environment, it is imperative that you prepare for each visit. If it is the first time you are seeing a doctor, you need to do all of the preparation in this chapter, plus a few more things. Go to the office with your family health history, a complete medical history, and a complete list and dosages of all the prescription drugs you are taking along with all vitamins and herbal supplements. You should maintain all of these records on an ongoing basis for yourself anyway and have a copy for any new doctor. Be prepared to explain any new symptom or change in your condition to your doctor. It's good to make notes on how often these occur, the severity, and the length, times of day, and what you are

---

DOCTOR VISIT CHECKLIST

- ◆ List of medications and doses plus vitamins and supplements
- ◆ Details on any new symptom or change in condition
- ◆ List of questions ready for the doctor
- ◆ Daily chart of blood sugar readings (diabetics)
- ◆ Write names and dosages of new prescriptions in your notes
- ◆ Ask questions about new prescriptions

doing when the symptoms occur. The better you can explain the symptoms to your doctor, the more likely the doctor can accurately diagnose your problem.

Have a list of questions prepared with the most important ones listed first. You can even have a copy of the questions written out for your doctor and give it to him when you first see him.

HEART POINT

WARNING: Do not talk while your doctor is writing a prescription. A tiny error could be deadly: a misplaced decimal point, number of pills per day, or even one letter. One letter misplaced can spell out tragedy.

During the visit, write the name and dosage-amount of new prescription medicines in your own notes. You can then double check your notes against the medicines you get from the pharmacy. This can help prevent errors. We can't read our doctor's handwriting and don't want to take the chance that the pharmacist can't either.

Ask questions about the new prescriptions, about the doses, side effects, and efficacy. You should always ask, "What will this medicine do for me?" or, "Why are you prescribing that?" This may only be the beginning of the process, but you need to understand the medicines you are taking. Get all of the information you can from your doctor. Try to understand why he is prescribing this particular medicine to you now.

DARRELL'S STORY

"Nearing the end of a visit with my cardiologist, shortly after my bypass surgery, I noticed him reaching for his prescription pad and starting to write. I stopped him and asked what he was prescribing for me. He replied that he was giving me something for my heart rate; it was a bit elevated. I explained that this must be some short-term aberration as I monitor my resting heart rate and it is generally around sixty beats per minute. He said that level is fine and that we would just continue to monitor it in the future. He didn't finish writing that prescription and I have never had to take anything for my heart rate. Being aware of your own body and being assertive can prevent taking unnecessary medications."

Take notes with a pencil and pad you bring to each appointment. If you can't do it in the exam room, or have someone do it for you, take a moment before you leave and make notations in the waiting room. Make certain you know and understand what the doctor told you and any medical terms she used. Ask for clarification before you leave the office.

CATHY'S STORY
(caregiver, 50)

"My dad was put on a blood thinner medication and had been on it for three to four weeks. No one told him that he should have regular check-ups the first month he was on it. He started having problems and was bleeding into his eye. When I saw him, his eye was completely red and the blood had run down and caused him to have a horrible black eye. I started asking him about his diet and medication and discovered he was eating large amounts of food containing vitamin K, which was normal for him, but a bad combination with the medication. I had him call his doctor and go in immediately."

Dealing with Doctors

The rule of mutual respect applies to doctors as well as patients and caregivers. If you treat your health professionals with respect and patience but do not receive the same treatment in return, look somewhere else. A doctor or staff member who is genuinely concerned with patients and caregivers will exercise consideration and respect as much as possible. Any doctor who has the best interest of the patient in mind should be open to a second opinion to make sure the patient is receiving the right recommendations and treatments. If you feel that a doctor isn't meeting your expectations, express concerns, and if no improvement follows, find another doctor.

ELLEN'S STORY

"My dad was having some problems and went to his internist, who recommended he go see a cardiologist. As it turned out, Dad was experiencing congestive heart failure. The cardiologist ordered a procedure and then put my father on medication. My parents were new to the world of heart problems and did not know what questions to ask. When Dad started experiencing problems, Mother called the doctor's office only to be told that the doctor would be out of town for two weeks. She found the office staff and nurses unsympathetic and at no time did they tell her that she could call one of the other doctors in the office and get help. Neither the cardiologist nor his staff went the second mile to make sure my parents knew exactly what was happening, what the medication would do, and how to get further questions answered. I insisted that they call the internist and get some answers and get another referral. They were hesitant. It's hard to change doctors.

"When my dad ended up in the emergency room, my mother told their internist that she did not want him to call the same cardiologist. He recommended another one, who has turned out to be the perfect match for my parents. The doctor–patient relationship could not be better. Not only do they trust his medical judgment, but he also takes the time to genuinely show that he cares about them and about their concerns. They have talked to others who use him and to others who work in the hospital, and everyone talks about what a kind and caring doctor he is. When he decided to change hospitals this past year, he told my parents that he would recommend another doctor to them if they wanted to stay with the same hospital. They emphatically said, 'NO! We will change hospitals with you!'

"After using the same hospital for over forty years, they were willing to change because they found a doctor who was medically competent and knew that the total health and well-being of his patients makes a difference. In addition, his nurses and office staff reflect the same professional expertise and concern every time my parents make a visit or need to get their questions answered."

In Star Point Two, we discussed some terms you will hear health professionals use in conjunction with heart disease. At some point the doctor will talk about treatments and medications. Staying informed and keeping up with appointments, terms, medicine, and rehabilitation programs are all crucial to the patient's ongoing health. Doctors should not be the only source of medical information. You and your patient can get information from your pharmacist, patient support groups, a cardiac rehabilitation program, national medical organizations, books, magazine and medical journal articles, and the Internet (only from trusted sources/doctors with references).

Keeping Up

We suggest that you keep a large monthly calendar at the patient's home and at the caregiver's home if it's a different location. Record: Doctor (medical, ophthalmologist, dentist, etc.) appointments, scheduled lab work, and prescription renewal dates. Also record other significant dates, such as parties, due dates for bill payments, travel, pet appointments, and hair salon appointments. Having all these on the calendar ensures that you help to reduce stress in keeping up with personal commitments.

At the beginning of each month, or each week if needed, review the dates. If both patient and caregiver know about the doctor appointments, it can help create a checks and balances system to make sure all questions get answered. The caregiver can give input on questions to ask, and after the visit, the patient can provide an update.

Both patient and caregiver need to keep pocket or purse calendars with them at all times. Make sure dates on your pocket calendars match dates on home calendars.

Both patient and caregiver should keep a journal record of the patient's physical and emotional changes. This will prove invaluable in the future. Tracking when symptoms change and occur can help you see if a medication is working right or causing additional problems. Watching for behavior changes can indicate if certain procedures or stresses affect the patient's emotional well-being.

The caregiver and patient should keep a list of the patient's medications and doses with them at all times, in case of an emergency. Fold it to fit in a billfold or purse. The patient and caregiver need to communicate regularly to keep the list current. Include medications along with any vitamins or supplements.

Your Medical Records

It is important to track your own medical history. In Star Point One we showed you how to create your family medical history. In addition to that, you should create your own, in-depth personal medical history, plus an ongoing record of all your doctor visits, procedures and tests, laboratory tests and results, surgeries, medications, and nonprescription drugs and supplements. In some states, you are legally entitled to copies of all your medical records, including your doctor's charts and hospital charts. Most of the time, your own complete records will be more useful to you. Charts are written in "medical shorthand" and are filled with abbreviations that are difficult to decipher. It is certainly easier to maintain your own ongoing records. The other significant advantage to this is that through the process of collecting and recording you will increase your knowledge of the medical procedures and results of laboratory tests. You will be better prepared to follow up with your doctors or to know when you should do additional research.

Your Insurance

Patients and caregivers also must be aware of how to manage insurance or health maintenance organization (HMO) coverage to get the maximum benefit. It gets more difficult each day to work through the maze of restrictions insurance companies and HMOs place on their policyholders. You can learn about your coverage by examining existing policies, getting help if necessary. With that higher level of understanding, choices can be made for maximizing benefits. You also need to know your appeal rights, both what the organization gives you by contract and others you have by state or federal law. At this time state laws tend to have more protection for consumers than federal law. There is much political pressure to change these laws, so stay up to date. Be as tough as necessary to get the coverage you need. A threat to go to the state commissioner of insurance often gets action from companies. If all else fails, you may need to involve a patient advocate or an attorney.

FIND THE BEST HOSPITAL

YOU NOT ONLY need to understand what is happening to your heart, you need to carefully select where to have invasive tests or surgery. Patients and caregivers need to think through this process and carefully select a hospital and surgeon. In this section we give you guidelines to help choose a hospital. Some of the considerations include the hospital's reputation, specialties, and medical staff.

A hospital's reputation is built through its history, both the length of time it has been in operation and the quality of care it provides. There are independent assessments of hospitals such as the *U.S. News and World Report* annual report of the "best" hospitals in the United States. They rank hospitals using a specific set of criteria. There are also the published mortality figures for your specific operation. In this book, that usually means a bypass. Keep in mind that a hospital with a very low mortality rate may take only take low-risk patients. Some hospitals have a reputation for tackling the most difficult of cases, those expected to have a lower success rate. That difference will be identified by talking to medical professionals, your primary care doctor, your cardiologist, and others. You also want to find out which hospitals are forward thinking and using the newest techniques (you may not want to try one of those, preferring the tried-and-true methods). Those hospitals will be among the first to perfect the newest operations. The hospital's reputation with the medical community and patients is also a valid guide. Find out where nurses or other doctors would go if they or a member of their family needed heart surgery.

DARRELL'S STORY

"I spoke to many people who had heart surgery, listened to their experiences, and got their recommendations on hospitals and surgeons. I was lucky that in the New York City area there are a number of very high quality hospitals and surgeons. I worked with that short list and found out which hospitals where covered by my insurance plan. I then selected surgeons at covered hospitals and 'referred myself' for additional opinions. I described this process to friends as interviewing the surgeons. These extra consultations or second and third opinions may not be covered by your insurance company. I decided they were important and went through the process anyway. One of those additional consultations cost me $500, but it was worth it. It was all part of me being in charge. I listened as the surgeons analyzed my case and I asked additional questions. With a lot of research about bypass surgery prior to those meetings, I was able to make a more educated choice of surgeon."

A hospital's specialty is important. You want a hospital that specializes in heart surgery or one that, at least, does a large number each year. Research suggests that hospitals that do a large number of a particular operation tend to have the best results. Recent research, detailed in the December 1, 2001, issue of the *Journal of American College of Cardiology* shows the mortality for bypass surgery was 1.99 percent for high-volume centers (more than 200 cases per year) and 3.3 percent for lower-volume centers. The study's authors suggested that it is very important for higher risk and severely at-risk patients to have surgery in the high-volume centers.

Hospital Education

Many hospitals that perform heart procedures offer educational information and presentations for patients, caregivers, and family members. *Don't* skip it. You will receive information about the hospital's cardiac rehabilitation program and find out about support groups. Some hospitals show a video explaining heart procedures and follow-up care or send a video home with the patient for future reference. In addition to receiving information, you will meet other patients and caregivers and know that you are not alone in what you are facing. Marilyn Walker, a cardiac physician's extender, says, "The hospital education program helps both the patient and caregiver. We send a video home with the patient because we know it is hard for anyone in that situation to absorb all the information the first time. The video and materials allow them to go back and review. We really push a healthy lifestyle in our program. A dietician talks to the group and we introduce the patients and caregivers to the hospital cardiac rehab program. We try to tell the patient about the unexpected things that might happen and cause alarm. If the group hears that patients might have hot flashes for a few weeks or their chest bone will make popping noises, they are more prepared when it happens."

DISCUSS SURGICAL OPTIONS WITH YOUR DOCTORS

IT IS OFTEN difficult to calmly discuss the possibility of having bypass surgery or other options with your doctor. Ideally you will have some time to do research and talk to several doctors with diverse opinions. You want to know if you really need the surgery or if there are alternatives. There are doctors who strongly support surgical choices and others who support lifestyle improvements. Ask your surgeon the following:

- ◆ What are my alternatives to the surgery?
- ◆ What is likely to happen if I choose the alternative?
- ◆ What is likely to happen if I do not have the surgery?
- ◆ In what ways is this surgery dangerous?
- ◆ Are there common complications with this surgery?
- ◆ What are my odds of having a stroke?
- ◆ What is my likelihood of having neurological complications?
- ◆ How often have you performed this surgery this year?
- ◆ What is your (the national, the hospital's) complication and mortality rate for this surgery?
- ◆ What is the mortality rate for patients of my age and condition?
- ◆ How long will it take me to recover?

This list also sums up the core of *informed consent.* In the past, doctors simply made decisions for patients and proceeded with the treatment they felt was best. Now, by law, doctors must inform you about their proposed treatment, options, risks, and benefits of alternative treatment. Prior to surgery, you will be asked to sign a form saying that you understand what the doctor will do and that you agree to it. Get a copy of the informed consent form ahead of time. Read it carefully and make sure you understand what it says and what you are agreeing to.

Weighing the Benefits and Risks of Bypass Surgery

Bypass surgery has become the accepted treatment for a wide range of patients with an equally wide range in severity of heart disease. There were 70,000 procedures done in 1972. *The New York Times* reported a recent estimate of over 600,000 procedures. Is the increasing number of procedures justified and for which patients?

A group of patients who clearly benefit from bypass surgery are those with a blockage in the left main coronary artery, especially those who also have reduced function of the left ventricle. The left main coronary artery is the one-inch-diameter artery that branches into the left anterior descending artery and the left circumflex artery. A blockage in this artery is extremely dangerous because it supplies the vast majority of blood to the left side of the heart. An early and important study of 686 patients in Veterans Administration hospitals showed clearly that patients with a blockage in the left main coronary artery benefited from bypass surgery. After three years, about 82 percent of those who had surgery survived verses 34 percent who were treated medically.

> "When I decided to have the bypass I wasn't sure that it would extend my life, but I knew it would allow me to live my life to the fullest."

Another group of patients who benefit are those who have incapacitating angina that has not been alleviated with proper medical treatment. A bypass will reduce pain for those patients and allow them to resume a normal life.

For the balance of patients, those who did not have a blockage in the left main coronary artery, there was no conclusive evidence that the survival rate improved or that the number of heart attacks decreased compared to those who did not have surgery. Research from the best heart centers, which do the highest volume of bypass surgeries, does show more positive results than studies of randomly selected patients. This is encouraging for those who select one of the top centers as the location for their surgery.

Another important study, the Coronary Artery Surgery Study (CASS), was funded by the National Heart, Lung, and Blood Institute and described in the November 1983 issue of *Circulation*. In the late 1970s, 16,626 angiogram patients were screened from eleven hospitals. Seven hundred eighty patients were selected to represent a range of significant blockages in one, two, or three major arteries. Each patient had stable angina and good heart function. Half of these patients had conservative treatment, half had surgery. The published results showed that surgery offered no improvement in longevity or number of heart attacks over those treated with medication, though it did relieve pain and gave patients a less restricted lifestyle while taking fewer prescribed drugs. Even for patients with triple artery disease, the results are mixed, though most surgeons seem to recommend the operation and survival rates are somewhat higher than for those treated medically.

A recent study compared bypass surgery to angioplasty with stenting in patients with multivessel heart disease. The article published in the *New England Journal of Medicine* showed little difference in rates of stroke, heart attack, or death for patients in both groups after one year. More time will be needed to show any differences in the long term. One group of patients, diabetics, has a much lower success rate with angioplasty than do other groups.

Some of the considerations that are part of the decision to recommend bypass surgery include the intensity of your angina (how much pain) and whether it is unstable or stable angina. Unstable angina indicates a greater chance of a heart attack. Another issue is how many arteries are blocked and what locations are included. Some blockages are much more dangerous than others. Other considerations are your age, general health, and other problems such as carotid artery disease, diabetes, and lung disease.

You need to weigh carefully your alternatives. Bypass surgery is major surgery with risks. Learn all the possible benefits along with each risk. Get a second opinion, at least. Surgical techniques continue to improve at a rapid pace. You need the most up-to-date information and options.

Every patient and case of heart disease is unique. The bias in the system is for action. Surgeons are good at surgery and know they can help patients using it. There is also a likelihood that fear of lawsuits causes doctors to err on the side of recommending surgery. Some doctors—Dr. Dean Ornish and others—believe you can reverse closed arteries with a lifestyle of exercise, low-fat eating, and stress reduction. Even they don't believe that it works for every situation, but patients need to know that research shows that these lifestyle approaches can reverse lesions in arteries for many patients. Others suggest medical management with drugs until the pain becomes unbearable.

HEART POINT

Bypass surgery provides symptomatic relief; it may not lengthen your life.

Often the choice becomes one of quality of life, as it was for Darrell. Even with triple artery disease, his prime motivator was dealing with the pain and restrictions on his life from the angina. "When I decided to have the bypass," Darrell says, "I wasn't sure that it would extend my life, but I knew it would allow me to live my life to the fullest." Be aware of all your options, work with the best professional medical personnel you can, and choose what is right for you and your lifestyle.

Surgical Risks

Heart–Lung Machine Problems

During most "open heart" procedures, a surgeon connects the patient to a heart–lung machine, which performs the functions of both the heart and lungs. Because the heart is "bypassed," no blood is pumping through it. The heart–lung machine takes the blood from the body, oxygenates it, and pumps it back into and through the body. All organs, except the heart, are supplied the life-giving blood.

To protect the heart, the body is cooled down and various chemicals are utilized to minimize the body's need for oxygen and to slow metabolism. This enables the surgeon to work on the heart that has stopped beating. Some surgeons now do what is called "beating heart" surgery, perhaps one of the most highly skilled surgeries of all.

DARRELL'S STORY

"I was concerned about the after-effects of the heart–lung machine during surgery. I wasn't afraid I would die—in fact, I was sure I wasn't going to—but losing mental ability was a real threat. I finally decided that I had selected one of the best hospitals and surgeons; it was now in the team's hands."

The heart–lung machine is a technological marvel that takes over the function of both organs to enable the surgeon to work on a nonbeating heart. Blood is diverted out of the body into the machine, where oxygen bubbles into the blood. It is pumped back into the body and, in reverse, through the body. These disruptions and changes in normal flow can dislodge cholesterol plaques, which may flow to other organs, including the brain. There may also be problems with specialized proteins that attack normal cells.

The potential damage is controversial. There are patients who experience some brain damage during surgery. An estimated 160,000 out of 400,000 bypass patients experience some loss in mental abilities. Some appear to be short-term losses, others longer-lasting or permanent. Because of the age of typical bypass patients, some or much of the loss may be linked to the aging process.

Many patients are confused for a time after surgery. Most cases seem to be only short term. An article in the *New England Journal of Medicine,* February 8, 2001, sums up and describes the breadth of the problem. It shows that from 33 percent to 88 percent of patients show some short-term cognitive decline after bypass surgery. There is also some risk of long-term brain injury from the machine. They also reported that 42 percent of patients showed cognitive decline five years after surgery. In most cases the decline was relatively "minor" and may be attributed to the age of the patients or to the surgery, the authors did not know. As this question is researched, more information will become available in the future. Discuss the issue with your doctor prior to surgery.

Other Surgical Risks

All surgery puts you at risk for several problems. Open wounds are susceptible to infection often spread by hand contact between hospital staff and patient. It helps to insist that staff wash hands before touching you. Also, request a room change if your roommate has an infection. It is also better to be shaved for surgery the morning of the procedure rather than the night before.

Even though anesthesia risks are relatively low, mistakes still can happen. These are usually caused by human error. Protect yourself by knowing who the anesthesiologist is, what training he or she has, and if he or she has been sanctioned.

There are potential errors during surgery such as the surgeon cutting nearby tissue by accident or leaving a sponge or other equipment inside your body. There are also risks of just being in the hospital. Of particular concern is medication error. The best protection is to know what has been prescribed by your doctor, the amounts, and what it looks like. You can ask what each medication is before you take it, or better yet, be able to identify your medicines.

DARRELL'S STORY

(Bypass Surgery: 10/20/98)

BEFORE THE SURGERY

"After I had made my choice of surgeon, Dr. Bercow, and St. Francis Hospital, I selected a date for my procedure. I was finishing my book *Kitchen Garden Planner*, and the writing would be done on a Sunday. I called to make my appointment and told them the week I was available. They offered the following Monday. I turned it down and requested midweek and settled on a Tuesday. (I doubt that it really is like not wanting to purchase a car that was produced on Monday, but it made me feel better.) Soon after making the appointment, I attended, along with other patients and many of their caregivers, a presurgery class at the hospital. It was terrific. We were told what would happen before, during, and after the surgery. I particularly remember being encouraged to plan something 'big' after the surgery. We were told that about 40 percent of our recovery was mental and those who go into surgery with a positive attitude recover more quickly.

"The surgeon's office sent a list of instructions: what medicines to stop taking before surgery (blood thinners) and a suggested list of vitamins and supplements. I was already taking all of them, including coenzyme Q10.

DAY I

5:30 AM "I arrived at St. Francis Hospital. I was a little late as traffic was surprisingly heavy. I drove. I wasn't nervous. I was prepared; I had researched the issues, talked to people, worked through it, made decisions, and controlled everything I could. I filled out the Health Proxy to give instructions if I became incapacitated.

6:30 AM "I moved up to the prep area. A group of nurses started working on me. They shaved my body from ankles to my neck. The anesthesiologist came in, introduced himself, asked me questions, and started putting in IV lines, etc. The Foley catheter and breathing tube would be installed after I was under anesthesia. He gave me something to relax me. My surgeon, Dr. Bercow, came in. He talked to me more about the surgery in a reassuring manner. I didn't have any more questions. He then asked me about using the artery from my arm instead of my leg. I basically said, 'I already decided to trust you; you can make that call.'

8:30 AM "They rolled me into the operating room. There were two or three people working, dressed in scrubs. I remember thinking how tall everyone was. Maybe it was the angle, but I don't think so. I thought about the studies that showed tall people were more successful than others. I also wondered if they matched surgical teams by height as my surgeon is tall.

Later I saw one of the women on the team who was at least six feet tall. Then the anesthesiologist said I would feel some warmth, then . . . dreamland, well, asleep anyway and no memory of the actual surgery.

1:00 PM "I awoke in the recovery room. Nurses started talking to me and adjusting tubes and equipment. My wife came in to see me. She was surprised at how good I looked, after being warned how rough looking I might be. The respiratory therapist started talking to me, asking me to do things. Later, I realized he was working me through a protocol to wean me off the breathing tube. Within an hour, the tube was out. I was grateful. The tube was one of the worst parts. My throat felt like hell; I was very hoarse. Soon, I was trying to talk or croak out words. I asked the nurses for ice chips. I was able to feed them to myself. It was awkward with all the tubes and stuff in my arms and hands. You feel like a limp mummy. I could give myself pain medicine through the IV with the push of a button. I didn't feel any pain, so didn't exercise that option. I was feeling a little better and asked for something to drink, and the nurse brought me some ginger ale. They were special little short cans; I guess most patients don't drink much. I drank the first one, asked for another, drank that, and asked for more. I think I drank all of their ginger ale and decided to switch to water. First they gave me a cup of it, later a whole pitcher. They kept removing things from my body and I kept talking. It was very busy, lots of patients coming out of surgery with many things to do for each one. I was the most alert patient in there. They talked about getting me out of bed. I'm unclear if it was my surgeon's instruction or suggestion; I knew it was unusual.

10:00 PM "Things seemed to calm down in the room. There was also a partial shift change. They talked about getting me out of bed again. It took three of them. It was a very complicated operation, wires, tubes, and the bulk of my weak body.

11:00 PM "I'm finally sitting in a chair and continue to observe the activity around me. I continue talking to the nurses. I am very awake, almost wired with excitement.

DAY 2

2:00 AM "I tell the nurses that I should try to sleep. They reversed the complicated moving operation and got me back in bed. I asked for something to help relax me and go to sleep.

5:30 AM "I awaken at my normal time and am soon fully alert. There is more talking, more tubes to pull out, and a discussion about moving me to a regular room. I continue to observe the action throughout the room. I feel sorry for a man who is having problems with breathing and the tube. He still had the tube in twenty-four hours after his surgery. I stayed awake, not even drowsy.

9:00 AM "I am feeling pretty good. The nurses kept checking my comfort and pain level. I never really was in pain. I never used the morphine button. They asked if I wanted breakfast. I did, I was quite hungry. I got to choose between a liquid breakfast and something between liquid and solid. I chose the 'between.'

10:30 AM "My breakfast of farina, yuck, a roll, cold cereal, and 1-percent milk arrives. I recall how the milk tasted like ice cream (I had been using only nonfat milk for some time.) At the same time, space was becoming an issue. More patients were coming out of the OR who needed lots of help and no bed open for me yet. The nurses continued to juggle. They told me a bed was open and called someone to move me. My original respiratory therapist came and noted that I was 95 percent (oxygen saturation in my blood) on room air. He wondered what I was still doing there and joked, 'Get the hell out of here; we need this bed for sick people.' We laughed. I was feeling good and not like a sick person.

11:00 AM "They rolled me down to room 380. The OR and recovery room were on the third floor but in a different wing of the hospital. I remember the safety grids across the sloping hallway. They put me in a regular hospital bed. The nurse seemed surprised at how good I looked for coming from the recovery room. I felt good. I was going to take the suggested pain medication. That recommendation was to preempt the possibility of pain so that I wouldn't hesitate to get out of bed and walk. Another nurse came in and asked me some questions. 'What is your name?' 'What day is it?' 'Who is the president?' The first two were no problem, but on the third I had to stop and think. I wished I would have read that brochure more closely; who is the hospital president? Then I laughed to myself and answered, 'Bill Clinton.' These were not meant to be complicated, just simple questions to see if I had lost any mental ability after the surgery.

11:45 AM "When she finished with the questions (I think I passed), I told her I would like to walk. A nurse's aide came in and helped me out of bed and we started to walk. She seemed surprised at my strength, yet she didn't want me to overdo it. I walked around the corner and then to the next corner. Heart markers were on the floor at twenty-foot intervals so you could keep track of your progress. I think I walked a hundred feet the first time. I felt I could do more but didn't want to be stupid, so turned and went back to bed.

12:15 PM "I rang for help and asked to walk some more. One of the rules you agree to when you move into this section of the hospital is to not get out of bed without help. By that time I had become the star patient and got lots of encouraging comments from the nurses.

12:45 PM "My wife arrives. She had gone to the recovery area at the designated visiting hours because my move hadn't been picked up by the hospital computer and I couldn't reach her by phone. I had called my family and editor. They were very surprised to hear from me so soon and then relayed information to others. I wanted to walk again and asked the nurse if I could walk with my wife this time. She said yes, but she would be jealous. The flattery from a young, cute nurse improved my spirits some more. I got up and did a few laps around the nurses' station, getting some more encouraging comments.

"Later I asked permission to get up on my own. Using a urinal sucks. So, within about thirty hours of when my surgery ended, I was able to get in and out of bed and go to the bathroom on my own. That was a big deal. I think I slept five hours that night, a little less than normal. That also took a little negotiation with the nurse about my medications, one that they would have to wake me up to give me. I explained my normal pattern with my medications and suggested that moving the chart schedule by an hour and letting me sleep would be better all around. She agreed.

DAY 3

"I felt great; I remember getting up and walking four times during the day. Each walk was for at least a quarter-mile, probably more. The heart markers were at twenty-foot intervals, but the corners seemed to present some measurement problems. They weren't used to patients doing laps. I figured it was about fourteen laps around the nurses' station. So, I literally walked more than one mile the second day after my surgery. By the time the assigned cardiologist (my personal cardiologist did not have privileges at the hospital) showed up, I was pretty tired. I really did not have the level of fatigue that I was told to expect. He commented on my walking, but I guess I looked tired by then. He said that I might be out by Sunday. I knew he was wrong. I felt like I could have gone home that afternoon. I felt good enough, though I had no clue about potential problems, like infection or others. After he left, I asked the nurse to let my surgeon know about my progress.

DAY 4

"I felt great in the morning, maybe a little upset because of the cardiologist saying I might have to stay. I decided I was going home. I walked a bit, maybe not as much as the day before. Maybe I was saving my strength to deal with the doctor. I got up to walk around noon and strolled around the corner. My surgeon, Dr. Bercow, was sitting at the nurses' station talking to a nurse. He looked up and said, 'I hear you want to go home.' And I said, 'Sure.' I think he said, 'Okay' and reached for a release and filled it out. He reminded me to slowly increase my activity level and joked that I probably wouldn't be up to tennis right away. I called my wife, Geri, who was working that day, and told her to come and get me. She started juggling her schedule; she was not expecting me to be released so soon, and was there at about 5:00 PM I made a point of showing her, with the nurse present, the spot on my chest that was still oozing slightly. That was where the drain tube had been. I didn't want her to panic, and to know that I was really fine. We left the hospital and she drove home using a route by the Lord & Taylor department store. (Why do you suppose women use stores as landmarks?) We went through the drive-through at Wendy's and ordered our favorite low-fat meal: chicken Caesar pita (no longer available) with no dressing. We use the no-fat dressing at home. We ate and soon became tired, going to bed at about 9:00. A typical stay for a standard bypass is from five to seven nights. I had spent only three nights in the hospital—a remarkably short stay."

GIVE SUPPORT AFTER THE SURGERY

Helping the Patient Survive the Hospital Stay

If you have ever watched a beauty pageant, you know the speech. The first runner-up never knows when she might be called on to take over. Neither does an understudy. When a cast is chosen for a production, understudies are chosen for the principal roles. An understudy is someone who knows the role and has the acting ability to step in if something happens to the principal performer.

It would be careless and selfish for a caregiver to sit back and not learn all he or she can about heart disease in case the need arises to step in and manage the team when the patient cannot. If you are a caregiver, you can't get answers while you are crying and waiting for someone else to do the asking. If your patient is incapacitated, then you have no choice but to "step up to the plate" and take control of the situation. Before anything is done "to your patient," you have the right to know why and what results are expected. Do not let one medication be given or one procedure be done without getting the information you need.

In what areas should you make certain you receive accurate information? Following are some important questions for which you should seek answers.

Problems

♦ What damage occurred?

♦ Can it be reversed?

♦ What caused it?

♦ Will it happen again?

Procedures

♦ Why is the procedure or surgery needed?

♦ What are the expected results?

♦ What are the risks?

♦ Are there any other options?

♦ How long is the recovery period?

Prognosis

♦ What changes need to be made in the patient's lifestyle?

♦ What ongoing medical care is necessary?

♦ When can the patient resume routines?

Medications

♦ Why is the medicine necessary?

♦ What are the desired results?

♦ What are the risks and side effects?

♦ How long will the patient have to take the drug?

♦ If you or the patient has a concern about the medication, what is the procedure to get questions answered as quickly as possible? *(We provide in-depth information about managing medication in Star Point Four.)*

Support

♦ Are there materials we can read to learn more?

♦ Are there support groups in our area?

♦ Do you recommend the hospital's rehab program?

After a medication is administered or a procedure done, watch your patient closely. Many hospitals are understaffed, and it's impossible for them to check on your patient and note every change that occurs. Plus, you know your patient better than they do. Marilyn Walker, R.N., is a physician's extender for a cardiologist. She works with patients and families in pre-op education and follows them throughout their hospital stay. Marilyn contends that, unfortunately, the nurse–patient ratio is not always what it should be. Most of her patients handle the hospital experience better if a family member or friend stays with them. "It not only helps the patient's attitude, but ensures that someone is checking on them around the clock." Marilyn sees patients with a support system and a strong belief or faith doing the best in the hospital.

Keep a running list of your patient's physical and emotional behavior, and when a nurse routinely comes in the hospital room, give an update. You don't have to be a pain about it. Simply give the nurse the information. Write down the name of any medications being given and know how much is being administered and how often. Some nurses and doctors might seem bothered if they have to stop and spell a medication for you or tell you its purpose. Let them. You are paying them for their expertise and service. There is no rule book that says the doctor cannot tell you the name of a medicine or the side effects of a procedure. So keep on asking. This is not like building a house. If a mistake is made or something left out, a builder can tear the house down and start over. But this is someone you love and their life is at stake.

Heads Up for Caregivers

We didn't say it would be easy to be the one in control. Each person's circumstances are different. But after interviewing patients, caregivers, doctors, and nurses, we found some common occurrences. Knowing about them will help you become more aware and perhaps deal with a situation better so that you reduce your stress load.

While your patient is incapacitated, someone will have to supervise the flow of traffic. What do we mean?

♦   There will be overbearing relatives and friends who have good intentions but are not considerate of the patient's stamina level during recovery. Many caregivers tell unfortunate stories of visitors who came to the hospital and stay and stay. The hospital staff cannot possibly monitor every visitor and how long he or she stays. It will be the caregiver's responsibility to tell visitors when they can stay and when they should go. We suggest that you find another friend or relative who can help. As a caregiver you will have enough to do watching and caring for the patient and for yourself.

ELLEN'S STORY

"When my dad had bypass surgery, my mom was completely focused on him and his recovery. I 'kept watch.' If Dad had been experiencing pain or discomfort or was resting, I would not let visitors come in. I could not believe how forceful I had to get with some of them. I know they cared about my father, but their presence was not what he needed to get better while in the hospital. I had to sit by the phone to catch all the calls. It amazed me that people felt they had to call his room to check on him. They wanted to be supportive, but often were disruptive. After he got home and was recuperating, visitors were welcomed as his strength increased."

♦   The doctors and nurses will not be there every moment. Know that you can press the call button for the nurse or scream out and someone will come quickly if there is an emergency. If your need or question is not specifically urgent, then it might take a little while for someone to get to you. Try to think ahead about pain medication and keep up with when your patient should get it again. Remember to note any changes (good and bad) to report to nurses and doctors.

♦   Although it will be difficult for you to leave the bedside of your patient, you will need to do so to get extra clothes, or to eat, or to go home and take a nap, or simply to take a break. Walking away for a period of time is not only okay, it is highly recommended. If you allow yourself to become emotionally and physically depleted in the hospital, you will be in no shape to assist your patient when he or she comes home. Enlist someone you completely trust to sit with the patient while you are away. If you do want visitors to come in until you return, make certain you tell the person staying in your place.

ELLEN'S STORY

"When either of my parents has been hospitalized and an immediate family member has not been able to be there, they have friends who always come and sit with them. One couple has a medical background, so my parents feel better leaving the hospital for a short time. I know that I can call the friends at any time to check on my parents."

Caregivers: Prepare to Manage

Both of us understand what it is like to be thrust into the world of medical terms, hospitals, doctors and nurses, and pharmacists. It can easily be overwhelming, especially when a patient's medical condition is critical. But, we could not throw up our hands and cry and wait to see what the doctors would do next. For Darrell, it was his own life; for Ellen, it was her father's life. Sitting back and letting someone else "hang in there for us" because we were scared and didn't want to bother the doctors or nurses would have been selfish and stupid. If you are a patient, *it is your life!* If you are a caregiver, *it is the life of someone you love!*

MAX'S AND MARIE'S STORY
(heart patient, 68) (caregiver, 67)

Max has always been the man in charge professionally and at home. He is a physically strong, big man. When Max was hospitalized and so critically ill he could not talk, Marie was devastated. She did not know what to do. The doctor would order medication, but Marie didn't know what it was supposed to do. Her husband had a procedure scheduled, but she wasn't sure why there was a waiting time. She spent much of her hospital stay worrying and crying to friends. She was scared to bring Max home.

ELLEN'S STORY

"My dad is a World War II veteran and has always been a strong, proud man. Even in ICU after bypass surgery, he was cracking jokes. When I visited him I asked him how he felt, and he said he wasn't going to run a race but felt just about like they told him he would. We were all much more concerned about his pain and recovery than he was. Because he is so strong, he doesn't like to say exactly how bad something hurts or give the details. Many times, my mother has had to describe the problem to a doctor or 'make' my dad go to the emergency room."

If you are not a person who deals well with change or uncertainty, dealing with heart disease will give you the opportunity to improve your skills! If you expect changes, especially in the first six months after a heart attack or surgery, then you will not be surprised when they occur. Give it time. Allow yourself and your patient to work through each change. Open communication and joint and individual outlets will keep you both sane while you work together to get through the tough times. Remember that you must take care of yourself so you can be the best caregiver for your patient. No one else will take care of you.

Recovery Phase

The average stay in the hospital after a conventional bypass is about a week, including at least one to three days in the Intensive Care Unit (ICU). For a minimally invasive bypass, estimate a three-to-five-day stay, though some patients return home after a day or two. Each patient is a unique case, so don't assume you will respond a particular way.

Everyone will recover at his or her own rate depending on many factors. Generally, you will be restricted in the amount of activity you can do. There are specific limits on what you can lift. You also must avoid any blow to the chest, which is why you are not allowed to drive for at least four weeks after the surgery. A car accident with your chest striking the steering wheel would be very bad for you. Other limits will be set by your doctors.

Caregiver Support

When the patient leaves the hospital, the caregiver will receive care instructions for the first phase of recovery. Usually the information is for the first eight weeks after surgery unless the patient has had a less invasive procedure. The information should cover the following areas:

Care of the incision
◆   Keep the incision clean and dry. Use only soap and water to clean it.

Signs of infection
◆   Call the doctor if you notice an increase in drainage from the incision, any opening of the incision line, an increase in redness or warmth around the incision, or if the patient has a temperature greater than 100.5 degrees Fahrenheit.

Managing pain
◆   The doctor will give you a pain prescription before the patient leaves the hospital. Get it filled immediately.

It is common for the patient to experience muscle or incision discomfort in addition to some itching, and feelings or tightness and/or numbness during the recovery time. If the pain reaches the level of what the patient experienced prior to surgery, call the doctor immediately. Many patients experience more pain in the arm or leg than in their chest if veins were grafted during surgery. Walking, performing regular activities, and time will gradually heal the leg or arm incision and decrease the pain, stiffness, and tightness.

If the patient is experiencing pain, encourage him to take medication about an hour before bedtime to enable him to rest better.

Monitoring activity level

♦ Ask the doctor any questions you have about the patient resuming activities at any time during the recovery period. During the first phase of recovery it is recommended that patients gradually increase their activity level. The patient should walk daily, following the instructions from the doctor, hospital educator, or cardiac rehab specialist. It is okay for the patient to climb stairs as long as it is not done repeatedly during the day or evening. Do not allow the patient to lift more than five pounds or to push or pull heavy objects during the first phase of recovery. The doctor will give you specific instructions about when the patient can drive again.

Changing sleep patterns

♦ Expect the patient to have some trouble sleeping for several weeks after surgery. For many patients, normal sleep patterns return in a few months, but others find they have to create new routines. If you notice that your patient's lack of sleep starts to interfere with her recovery or causes changes in behavior, call the doctor. Encourage the patient to report any changes in sleep patterns to the doctor at each visit. Patients should avoid caffeine in the evenings if they continue to have sleep problems. A gradual increase in activity and exercise helps many patients rest better at night.

Emotional changes

♦ After surgery, it is common for patients to feel depressed. If these feelings do not begin to lift after a few weeks or if they get worse, call the doctor. As a caregiver, you can help your patient improve by encouraging regular daily and weekly activities, including walking, hobbies, visiting with others, sharing feelings, resting, and participating in a support group and/or a cardiac rehabilitation program.

Diet instructions

♦ Don't be surprised if your patient has a poor appetite after surgery. Unfortunately, the appetite changes as healing progresses and soon you and your patient will need to make lifestyle changes in regard to eating habits. Star Point Five will give you excellent information about keeping your body healthy.

Depression

Depression following bypass surgery or a heart attack can be a significant problem. Many patients go through a short period of emotional readjustment after the surgery or a heart attack. If patients are down or have symptoms of depression for any length of time, they should seek help. The National Institute of Mental Health (NIMH) estimates that up to 20 percent of heart surgery patients who haven't had a heart attack and 40 percent to 60 percent of those who have had a heart attack suffer from depression. This problem can put a strain on friendships and marriages, even ending them. Depressed patients do not recover as quickly as others do. Depression can contribute to a worsening of symptoms and may affect adherence to treatment regimens. The NIMH suggests that those who have major depression after a heart attack are at a three to four times greater risk of dying within six months than those who don't have it. Anyone who has had problems with depression in the past should anticipate a problem and work with a professional before and after the surgery.

> ## HEART POINT
>
> After heart surgery, up to 20 percent of heart patients who haven't had a heart attack and 40 percent to 60 percent of those who have had a heart attack are estimated to suffer from depression.

If a patient has several of the following symptoms for more than two weeks, she should seek professional help:

- Eating disturbances: loss of appetite and weight, or weight gain
- Sleep disturbances: insomnia, early-morning waking or oversleeping
- Irritability
- Excessive crying

- ◆ Chronic aches and pains that don't respond to treatment
- ◆ Thoughts of death or suicide; suicide attempts
- ◆ Feelings of guilt, worthlessness, helplessness
- ◆ Difficulty concentrating, remembering, or making decisions
- ◆ Persistent sad or empty feeling
- ◆ Loss of interest or pleasure in ordinary activities, including sex
- ◆ Decreased energy or fatigue

Getting Back to Normal

DARRELL'S STORY

"I had cleared my calendar and had no plans for the month after my surgery. I had expected to lack energy and not be able to do much. The first morning at home I awakened at my normal 5:30 AM and went downstairs and made coffee (decaffeinated). I had been warned to plan my day on one level of the house as I would not be able to handle stairs. I felt much better than expected and was much stronger. I walked down the stairs to the basement and read e-mail and let everyone know how I was doing, 'Terrific!' I walked up the stairs and read the paper. When my wife, Geri, woke up I fixed her breakfast. I made pancakes, leaving out all the fat and eggs. They were awful (the new version of the recipe is in Star Point Five). In a few hours I was already getting fidgety and decided I would go for a walk. I didn't know how far I would feel like covering but started walking in quarter-mile out and back loops. I walked, slowly, about three miles. I was tired but elated. I was far more physically able than expected."

Plan on a slow return to normal activities. Your physical condition, age, and type and difficulty of the surgery will determine how fast you recover. Expect to be tired and unable to do much when you return home. For instance, if you live in a multistory house, plan your day to navigate stairs once in the morning and once at night. Your strength and endurance will build over time. In two to three weeks you will feel stronger and you will have more typical body habits again, such as appetite, sleep patterns, and bowel movements. Generally, if an activity does not cause fatigue it will be permitted.

Your doctor will give you an idea of the level of activity you may be able to do and specific limits you should not exceed. You are not allowed to lift anything that weighs more than five pounds. That includes groceries, grandchildren, and anything else you think of. You also are not allowed to drive for the first four weeks after surgery. The chest wall and rib cage need time to heal so they can protect the chest cavity in case of an accident.

If you work in an office, you can usually return to work in four to six weeks. If you do more physical work, it may take longer.

Patients and caregivers are often fearful about the patient resuming physical activities. It's good to discuss this and do some of these activities together. Try taking short walks together each day. Over time, strength and endurance build, as does everyone's confidence. Keep building your body back toward normal. After about four weeks ask your doctor to refer you to a cardiac rehab program (see more in Star Point Five), which will increase your physical abilities under supervision.

Sex After Heart Surgery

Generally, men and women can start having sex again within two to four weeks after angioplasty (with or without stents) and four to six weeks after bypass surgery or a heart attack. You can start again when you feel ready, but ask your doctor first. Sex takes about as much energy as walking up two flights of stairs. If you can do that comfortably, you can probably have sex.

> "Most people return to similar levels and types of sexual activity as before surgery or heart attack."

The physical changes you experience during sex gradually increase from mildly elevated breathing, heart rate, and blood pressure until the peak of orgasm. At the peak level the average heart rate is 115 beats per minute (ranges from 90 to 145 BPM) and blood pressure is up about 30 to 50 mm Hg. Soon after, your breathing, heart rate, and blood pressure return to normal levels. These are typical responses, including those people who have had heart attacks or surgery. Most people return to similar levels and types of sexual activity as before surgery or heart attack.

It is common after surgery or heart attack to experience some psychological barriers to a satisfying sexual life. Some people feel afraid, tired, sad, depressed, or less interested in life. Those feelings should go away soon, certainly within a few months. Seek help if they linger. The feelings can create havoc with resuming normal life and with your relationships.

Some patients and spouses worry that sex can cause a heart problem. This is not true, but if you have any doubts speak to your doctor about this. When couples have a satisfying sex life, other aspects of their lives are likely to improve at the same time.

It's good for couples to start to touch, snuggle, hold, and caress soon after returning from the hospital. You will feel comfortable and loved without the pressure to perform. With time, the comfort level continues to increase, and as energy increases you will both naturally move on to more vigorous activities. Generally, you will be able to resume intercourse about two to four weeks after angioplasty and four to six weeks after a heart attack.

As you resume or start a new healthy lifestyle, sex will naturally follow. Eating a healthy diet, getting exercise and plenty of rest, and taking medicines properly will make you feel more confident. Remember that some medicine can adversely affect sexual performance and desire (see Star Point Four). If you are taking new prescriptions for blood pres-

HEART POINT

Dr. Michael F. Roizen suggests in his book *Real Age* that people who have sex frequently can cut their "real age" by two to eight years. He suggest that having sex two times per week can add two years to your life and extrapolates other data to conclude that having sex and orgasms 350 times per year and a happy sex life (who wouldn't be) could add eight years to your life (practicing safe sex in a monogomous relationship). Sex is relaxing, cuts stress, and increases intimacy.

sure, irregular heartbeat, or chest pain, or diuretics, tranquilizers, and antidepressants, be vigilant to changes in desire or performance and discuss this with your doctor.

Anticipate Change

ELLEN'S STORY

"My dad always took care of everything that had to be fixed around the house and paid every bill. After his heart problems and his bypass surgery, my mom had to take over some of the responsibilities. After years of living with 'traditional' roles, my parents now understand how important it is to share responsibilities."

Understanding Changing Roles

With the onslaught of heart disease, all the individual and support roles are constantly changing. In the initial pre- and postsurgery hours, role reversal may quietly but aggressively begin. In some cases, the caregiver is thrust into the role of decision maker because the patient is too seriously ill to evaluate the situation.

DAUGHTER MELINDA'S STORY
(caregiver, 50)

"My mom, Margaret, had a heart attack and then had two angioplasties. After two years, the doctor said that her arteries were clogged again and she would need a triple bypass. I rushed around and got things ready to leave my family and drive the seven hours to be with my folks for the surgery. It took her several months to get her strength back. I thought I could stay for a week and then my father could take over being the main caregiver. When Mom didn't bounce back very quickly, he didn't know what to do. He doesn't really cook, and Mom always took care of the money and the shopping. He was retired and did pretty much what he wanted to most of the time. That changed when Mom had the surgery. He was so upset and worried that I ended up going back and forth for months. It was so hard to keep my work going, keep things going at my own home, and make the drive to help out. But I didn't have another choice. We didn't have money to pay for someone to come in and help, and they didn't really have friends who could help out very much. Little did I know that just when my dad was getting the hang of being supportive for my mom, we would face an even harder tragedy."

MOM MARGARET'S STORY
(heart patient, 74)

"I was scared to have the bypass surgery, but I thought I would get better as quickly as some other people I knew who had been through it. But I didn't. I couldn't get any energy back for a long time. I hated that Melinda had to keep coming up to help. I know it was so hard on her. And it was hard on my husband. He didn't really know what to do with me being sick. After the first year, he got better at helping with the grocery shopping and cleaning more. He even agreed to eat more healthy things with me. I think he would have finally come around, but he got sick and had surgery. As a result of the complications with the surgery, he died, and suddenly I was my own caregiver. It was the hardest thing I have ever been through for him to die. I guess I was kind of used to me being the patient and I was starting to lean on him more. Melinda had to start coming up again to help me sort through everything financially and go through all his things. I was taking a lot of nitro pills for angina. Melinda was worried about me at the same time she was dealing with her father's death. I don't know how we made it through all of it. Now she is my main caregiver. She comes up once a month or two months and checks all my medications with me and goes to the doctor with me. She wants

> "With heart disease, the role reversing can come and go over a period of years."

me to move down near her, but I just am not ready to give up my home here yet."

When illness and death strike, we take on roles we never thought we could handle. Spouses are called on to take on the role of husband and wife. Children are called on to parent their parents. Any time we go through a transition or a traumatic experience, it changes us. It is hard to see the changes while we are in the middle of it, but when the situation calms down or the pace slows down, it is good to stop and take stock of who you are, what you have been through, and how you want things to function in the future. After your patient is home and recuperating, take some time to sit and reflect. Sometimes situations occur so quickly that role reversal happens and patterns start developing that are not realistic and cannot continue. As you think about yourself as a caregiver and think about your patient, consider the following:

REFLECTIVE QUESTIONS FOR CAREGIVERS

We suggest you write down your responses to the following questions:

- How has your experience as a caregiver affected your life physically, emotionally, mentally, and spiritually?
- How has your role with your friend or relative changed?
- What is the most difficult challenge for you as a caregiver?
- Do you need to sit down and talk with the patient about the things that need to change?
- Do you need to talk with your own immediate family members to make some adjustments?
- Do you need to set up some routine appointments with a counselor to make sure you are dealing with everything and staying emotionally healthy?

Be a Team Player

You are there to support your patient as much as needed. If the need diminishes, then you must be willing to let go. Letting go doesn't mean your role is not important anymore. Look at it as if you are getting a reprieve from active duty. Renew your own energy so you will be ready if the situation changes. Celebrate that your patient is doing well and managing without your constant caregiving. Your loved one has moved from patient to parent, or partner, or friend again.

JAMES'S STORY
(heart patient, 66)

"After my wife died, my daughter assumed some of the role as a caregiver for me. As I worked through things and felt emotionally and physically stronger, it was hard for her to let go and let me take care of myself. It was even harder for her to let go when someone else came into my life."

One role reversal is hard enough, but with heart disease, the role reversing can come and go over a period of years. When there is a heart emergency, you become caretaker. When your patient starts recuperating again, you must move back to caregiver. It is hard not to become attached to your role at any given time.

Caregiver Traps

As roles change, watch out for caregiver traps that either you or the patient encounter.

Nurse

After your patient begins to recover, your role is to remind and encourage but not to be the nursemaid. Remind your patient to take her pills, but refrain from getting them out and putting them on the counter. Ask your patient what his blood sugar was, but don't stand over him while he takes it. Strongly suggest that your patient needs to slow down some or needs to call the doctor, but allow it to be his or her ultimate decision if it happens. Some patients will resent you playing nurse, while others will start depending on it. You don't want either situation. You want to move from being the team coach to just a team member. If you insist on being the coach, it will be all too easy for you to become a nagger.

Nagger

It is understandable that you care about your patient and want him to be as healthy as possible, but nagging is not a good means to an end. Eventually, you will build up resentment between you and your patient that will not be easily mended. The first couple of times you nag, results might occur. Your patient will take her pills or eat better for a while, but eventually she will sneak food or purposely not take her pills just because she wants to get away with it and do something you cannot stop her from doing. Nagging breeds resentment, which usually leads to anger. Anger adds stress to you and your patient's lives. Decide *not to nag!* Encourage, suggest, praise, and then let go. Ultimately, it is your patient's life and he must decide how to live it, no matter how much you worry.

Worrywart

If worrying could make your patient well or keep her from ever having heart problems again, then cardiologists would be out of business! Worrywarts get little else done except worrying because worry saps our physical and mental energy and becomes habit-forming. Worry becomes the caregiver's crutch to deal with situations and sometimes to get attention. But it seldom helps the patient and certainly adds stress to the caregiver. Refuse to become a worrier. Rely on your faith and on friends to support you. Gathering information will help you stay current with heart disease developments and give you a sense of empowerment that will reduce worry.

Don't Get Boxed In

When it comes to being a caregiver or caretaker, it requires that we step out of the box of what we imagined life would be like and allow it to be different. No one promised us that life would be easy. It is all about change and how we choose to handle it. Negative feelings and emotions will not make your situation or your patient any better. Choose to let the sides of the box down and change with the changes. To paraphrase the Recovery Prayer, "Change what you can and accept what you can't change."

There is overwhelming evidence that optimistic, well-adjusted people who are active in their communities and families live longer. Instead of thinking of your friend or loved one as a person with heart disease, think of him or her as a survivor. Every day your patient lives and functions, he or she is a survivor. And you are a survivor. Every day that

HEART POINT

Heart surgery gives nearly 5 million patients a year a second chance at life.

you live and function, you are a surviving caregiver. Take strength in the fact that you can face whatever comes because you have been through heart disease challenges before.

Author Susan Faughan examined the differences in optimists and pessimists in her work *Half Empty, Half Full: Understanding the Psychological Roots of Optimism.* Faughan contends that optimists trust that they can experience a range of emotions and not get "stuck." Pessimists don't really believe it's possible to change your state of mind; therefore, they don't believe they can trust themselves to handle any emotion and stay on an even keel. Which attitude toward life is going to help you the most as a caregiver? Which one will help you help your patient the most? It's up to you.

STAR POINT FOUR

Manage Your Treatment

PATIENTS MUST UNDERSTAND and be in control of their treatment. Caregivers need to be familiar with their patient's medications and with medical terms associated with heart disease. In this chapter we look at the various classes of drugs that a heart patient might take and types of surgery your doctor may recommend. We point out some of the virtually unlimited interactions of drugs with each other, with vitamin and mineral supplements, and with alcohol and food, along with providing information sources to enable you to investigate other combinations and tips for entirely new drugs. We want you to understand your medications, surgical options, and to be fully in charge.

DARRELL'S STORY

"I start each day by testing my blood glucose and then swallowing a handful of pills. They keep me alive, yet I know that a slipup or a misuse could kill me. These pills moderate or control my blood pressure, blood glucose, LDL and HDL cholesterol with a bonus pill, a low-dose antibiotic to help my gums stay healthy because the calcium channel blocker I use to control my blood pressure makes them worse—so many drugs that I need one to counteract the effects of another. I'm a chemistry experiment: multiple doctors and pharmacists all have a hand in my well-being and staying alive. I know that modern medicines can be miracle drugs or killers!"

Don't Let the Drugs Kill You

IT IS BEST to avoid overmedication. This is perhaps an obvious suggestion, yet an important one. If an improvement in lifestyle, a better diet, more exercise, and stress reduction can help you avoid adding even one more prescription drug to your daily routine, do that instead. This is the best way to take charge of your life and medicines.

Each new prescription drug adds a new level of complexity to the chemistry experiment that is your drug list. Each has the potential to interact with another drug you are already taking or interact with food you eat or drink or the vitamins you take for good health.

You should understand that doctors do not know the exact reaction that each new drug will have in/on your body or mind. Yes, they have a pretty good idea. They have scientific data from studies that tells them what is likely to happen. They judge the dose by your body weight and work with guidelines. But each new drug will work slightly differently in each patient. It can be somewhat more, or less, effective because of

> **"I know that modern medicines can be miracle drugs or killers!"**

your diet or even when or how you take the medicine. Doctors monitor patients who have started any new medications. Some medications require ongoing testing to judge their effectiveness and/or to test for side effects such as liver problems. You need to be aware of those issues and make sure you are tested at the proper interval.

Drug Basics

Know What You Are Taking

You should maintain a complete and up-to-date list of every prescription medication, herbal medication, vitamin and mineral supplement, and over-the-counter medication you currently take. A list of prescriptions that you formerly took should be a part of your personal medical history. For each new prescription, you should complete the Medication Question Guide that is provided later in this section.

"When my dad started seeing different doctors and getting so many prescriptions that he was running out of room in the medicine cabinet, I strongly suggested to my parents that they keep a list of his medications with them at all times. My mom now keeps a list of Dad's medications in her purse. She knows exactly what he is taking and tries to find out why he is taking it. On the day that he got out of the shower and his skin was turning black from his waist down, it was my mom who called the doctor and communicated the problem. The doctor knew immediately that my dad was having a reaction to one of his medications. Mom was familiar with the medication and its purpose. She was not disturbed when the doctor instructed my dad to stop taking the medication until his next appointment."

Caregivers, Ask and Ask Again

It is critical that the caregiver knows what the patient is taking and why. It did not surprise us to find out that medication was a top reason for confusion among the caregivers we surveyed. Remember the following tips when dealing with doctors and medication:

- You always have the right to ask questions.
- Doctors, nurses, and pharmacists can make mistakes. Always double-check what any health professional has told you. Repeat it back to them. Have the pharmacist check medication instructions against the doctor's orders if you have any doubts.
- Respect the life-stabilizing effect medication has on your patient, but do not let medications intimidate you. You can learn to pronounce their names and know why they are prescribed.
- Expect medications and dosages to be changed frequently, new med-

ications added, and others deleted. Understand how what time of day the medication should be taken, the amount, and how it will interact with other medications are determined in part by the patient's size, age, and medical problems. Don't expect your patient to be taking the exact same medications and doses that someone else you know is taking.

♦ If you and your patient approach the challenge of understanding and monitoring medication together, you will add strength to your total team. If you are both aware of any changes, it will be much easier when you visit the doctor to explain what effects the medicine has on you.

♦ Create an emergency plan if you or the patient notices serious side effects to any medication or treatment.

♦ Listen for complaints that could possibly be side effects such as dizziness, confusion, fatigue, depression, leg cramps, constipation, and nausea. Watch carefully when the patient starts a new drug or the dosage is changed.

The Bibliography and Resources include books, websites, organizations, and magazines that provide current information about heart disease, treatments, and medications.

JIM'S STORY
(heart patient, 66)

"I started out totally reliant on the medical folks. I just assumed they always knew what they were doing and what they were talking about. They never let on that they don't know something. But I began to see that they only knew about their specialty. I was taking nine different medications and feeling lousy. I took control of my medication. I sat down with each doctor and went over what I was taking and why and asked if I could drop some or try something else. I have cut back on several medications and been able to change some others.

"Cardiologists like to be artists. They love to draw the heart and show you how it is supposed to work. But my heart wasn't like every other heart. I felt like I was just another case to the doctors and surgeon. Taking control of my medications helped me feel like I knew what was going on with my body and my heart."

A Brown-Bag Checkup

The Institute for Safe Medication Practices suggests that you do an occasional "brown-bag checkup" for all the medications, supplements, and herbal medicines you are taking. This is particularly true if you have several doctors prescribing medicines for different chronic conditions. It also is true if you are changing doctors. Make an appointment with your primary care doctor, or the doctor who is your main "prescribing" doctor, to review all of your medicines, supplements, and doses you are taking. Put all of them in a "brown bag" or other container and take them to the appointment.

It is important that the doctor see everything you are taking. She also should know about anything that you take periodically. For instance, what is your favorite cold and flu remedy? Do you take mega-doses of vitamin C, echinacea, and zinc lozenges? Everything that you consume has a potential to interact with any of the drugs you are taking. Make sure your doctor knows about every one of them.

Review each of the medicines in the bag for dosages, frequency, and to determine if any medicine is outdated. This would be a good time for you to ask the doctor any questions you have about the medicines. If you have done some research before the appointment, you will be better able to discuss any issues you have.

Get Informed on Current Prescriptions

Every prescription drug has a manufacturer-produced package insert approved by the Food and Drug Administration (FDA). Get a copy for each prescription drug you take. Read and study them, and keep them in your personal medical file. Pay particular attention to the information on side effects and how and when to take the medicine. Review how much of each medicine is prescribed. Compare the manufacturer's recommendations to your doctor's instructions about when and how you should take it. If your doctor's instructions are different from the manufacturer's, call your doctor and discuss the problem. Confirm what each medicine looks like. The package insert will give you instructions on what to do if you miss a dose.

HEART POINT

WARNING: The patient information leaflets distributed by pharmacists are not regulated by the FDA and may be inadequate or misleading. Follow the advice in the FDA-approved package insert, particularly concerning drug interactions and side effects.

Over-the-Counter Medications

If you are thinking about using an over-the-counter medication, carefully read the entire label looking for ingredients that you should not take or that would cause you to have an allergic reaction. You need to know if they will react with any medications that you currently take. Ask the pharmacist and your physician for help and be certain that they know everything else you are taking.

Pharmacist Help

Try to use just one pharmacy. Select one that has a computer program that stores all of your prescription information and will check for interactions and allergies. Find out if they will also add your list of herbal supplements, vitamins, and minerals to their list.

Online Databases

There are now several online databases that can be used to check for interactions between drugs and between drugs and herbal medicines. These are listed in Resources. Use them for additional research.

Avoiding Drug Conflicts and Errors

Be sure to review your complete list of medications with each doctor at every visit. It's important to inform each doctor if a different doctor has changed your prescription medications in any way; the drugs, amounts, or how and when you take them. Perhaps the best way is to bring an updated list of all your medications and supplements to each appointment and to give it to the doctor.

HEART POINT

In the future, most doctors will use handheld computers to "write" prescriptions. This will eliminate errors in interpreting handwriting.

Don't talk to the doctor when she is writing a prescription. It is easy to make a small mistake in the amount of the drug, or even the spelling of a drug, if she is interrupted while writing. Confirm exactly what the doctor prescribed and how often you should take it. Write that information in your own notes. Compare this with the drugs you get from the pharmacy and make sure it is what was prescribed. Understand the purpose of the prescription and how long you will have to take it. Does it replace a medicine you are currently taking? What side effects are possible and what should you do about them?

Ask your doctor to write the purpose of the prescribed medicine on the prescription. With all of the look- and sound-alike drugs around, this is a double-check for getting what the doctor intended. It is also one more protection against a doctor's unreadable handwriting.

HEART POINT

Do not stop taking any medication suddenly. Always check with your doctor first.

If a doctor gives you any sample medications be sure to ask about their possible interactions with other drugs you are currently taking. You might ask your pharmacist to run a computer check of the sample drug against everything you are already taking. An alternative is to use the online databases, but you will probably have to run multiple checks to ensure the safety of combining the sample drug with all that you are currently taking.

JOHAN'S STORY

(heart patient, 55)

"A few months after my heart attack I was taking five or six medications. They caused problems with insomnia. I asked my doctor about them. He took me off three medications and cut the nitro in half. I slept and felt better."

Herbal Medicines

Just because something is natural or herbal does not make it safe. Many herbs and herbal remedies are extremely powerful, or even deadly, medicines. American consumers spend billions of dollars on herbs and supplements, frequently without discussing this with physicians. All herbal remedies need to be considered medicine and discussed with your doctors in order to avoid problems. Prior to surgery you should review your complete list of herbal medicines and supplements with the surgeon. Several common ones create dangerous problems for patients undergoing surgery. Ginkgo biloba and vitamin E thin the blood (garlic supplements are suspected of doing the same) and make clotting more difficult. These supplements, and all others, should be reviewed with your surgeon. Stop taking these seven days or more before surgery.

Take Medicine Exactly as Prescribed

Many people do not follow doctor's orders concerning prescriptions. Recent research reported in the July 2001 issue of the journal *Pharmacotherapy* indicates that of the individuals studied, almost 63 percent of those being treated for high blood pressure do not take their medicines correctly every time. This means that high blood pressure is not adequately controlled for nearly two-thirds of diagnosed patients. That puts them at significant risk for heart attack, stroke, and other avoidable problems.

HEART POINT

You cannot get "hooked" on blood pressure medication—take your medicine as prescribed.

Some of these patients forgot to take their prescription, but others knew they were supposed to take it but didn't because they thought they didn't need it or were worried about drug dependence, getting hooked on the drug. Patients should discuss these issues with their doctors.

HEART POINT

Phoning in a prescription can be dangerous. There are many sound-alike names for very different drugs. If your doctor does call in prescriptions, double-check the drug you receive with the name you have written down in the doctor's office or against the previous prescription.

Do not alter the form of any medication without your doctor's approval. Tablets and capsules should be taken exactly as they come from the pharmacy. Cutting tablets in half, or chewing or crushing them, may increase the rate they are absorbed into your body, make them ineffective or, even, make you sick.

Do not take anyone else's medicine or let anyone take some of yours.

Establish a Medicine Routine

To avoid problems taking your medications, establish a daily routine. Once you know when it is best to take each medicine, take it the same way at the same time each day. If you are confused, or the list is complicated, create a daily medicine list, with each medicine listed, with the dosage and time you should take it. Cross off each one as you take it. Once this list is created, make duplicates from a photocopier or a printer for your own records.

Store Drugs Safely

Handle your drugs like they are dangerous; they are. If children have any access to them, even during a short visit, keep your drugs in childproof containers or stored out of reach. Do not store your medicines with any that are prescribed for your pet. Dangerous mix-ups can occur. Also, do not store medicines in your bathroom medicine cabinet. They should be in a cool and dry location, out of direct sunlight, and not in the moist and warm conditions of your bathroom. It is best to store drugs in their original containers, or at least in containers that are carefully labeled. With labels, you can double-check exactly what you are taking. For the same reason, you want to take your medication in good light, certainly not in a dark room. This also avoids tragic mix-ups. Dispose of all outdated drugs and over-the-counter medications. Flushing them down the toilet is much safer than simply throwing them into the garbage, where curious kids and pets may find them.

Generic Versus Brand-Name Drugs

Drugs have several names. Ones with the same chemical structure, even if made by different manufacturers, would have the same generic name. Each of those products could also have a brand name. This is true for prescription and over-the-counter medications. A widely used example is aspirin, which is acetylsalicylic acid, the generic name. Brand names include Bayer, Anacin, and others.

There is a lot of disagreement in the medical community about taking a generic "equivalent" drug instead of a brand-name drug. Once the patent expires on a drug, other manufactures can produce their version of the same drug. Each generic drug should have the same amount of the active ingredient as the brand-name drug. The main differences, besides cost, are the bioavailability and quality, both difficult for a patient to weigh. Bioavailability describes how available the active ingredient will be to your body. Quality control defines how the drug is produced, stored, and dispensed by the manufacturer making the drug. Your pharmacist and doctor should be in a position to advise on these issues. Listen carefully to how they answer your questions about the drug. Do they say, "I think that for this specific drug it is better to stay with the brand name" and explain why, or, "This is the drug I always prescribe"?

HEART POINT

Sam had a difficult time swallowing some large pills. He has arthritis, so it is difficult to tip his head back quickly and move the pill to the back of his throat and swallow. He has found that he can easily take the pill by drinking the water through a straw. The directed water helps push the pill back and makes it easier to swallow.

In the first case, the doctor has thought through the issue and drawn a specific conclusion about this drug and its generic counterpart. The latter is a blanket statement.

What About You?

If you are a blood relative of a heart patient, you should be asking your doctor what kinds of medications or vitamins and supplements you should be taking. Each time a doctor prescribes a medication for you, inform him or her that you are at high risk for heart disease and inquire as to the effects of the medication on the heart.

TYPES OF CARDIAC DRUGS

THE SECTION THAT follows is a summary of some of the important drugs that doctors prescribe for heart patients. We provide a partial guide to side effects and possible interactions with other drugs, over-the-counter medications, food, and vitamin and herbal and mineral supplements. *This is not complete.* You need to be responsible and truly take charge of your medications; they really can kill you if not taken as prescribed. For each drug you are prescribed, do additional research online or in some of the excellent and detailed guides available. *Worst Pills, Best Pills* (by Sidney M. Wolfe, M.D.; Larry D. Sasich, Pharm. D., M.P.H.; Rose-Ellen Hope, R.Ph.; and Public Citizen Health Research Group) describes, in great detail, hundreds of good and bad drugs. More interactions between drugs, food, and supplements are described in Joe and Teresa Graedon's *The People's Guide to Deadly Drug Interactions.*

HEART POINT

Each year improper use of over-the-counter drugs results in 170,000 hospitalizations and costs about $750 million. (Source: White House press release, Office of the Vice President, March 11, 1999)

MEDICATION QUESTION GUIDE

Ask your health care provider these questions about each new medicine that is recommended or prescribed. Use a separate sheet for each medicine.

Name of Medicine _____

- ♦ What are the brand and generic names of the medicine? Can I use a generic form?
- ♦ What is the medicine for and what effect should I expect?
- ♦ Does this drug replace any other medicine I have been using?
- ♦ How and when will I use it, what amount will I use, and for how long?
- ♦ What do I do if I miss a dose?
- ♦ Should I avoid any other medicines (prescription or over-the-counter), dietary supplements, drinks, foods, or activities while using this drug?
- ♦ When should I notice a difference or improvement? When should I report back?
- ♦ Will I need to have any testing to monitor this drug's effects?
- ♦ Can this medicine be used safely with all my other medications and therapies? Could there be interactions?
- ♦ What are the possible side effects? What do I do if a side effect occurs?
- ♦ How and where do I store this medicine?
- ♦ Where and how can I get written information about this medicine? What other sources of information can I use to learn about this medicine?

Source: U.S. Food and Drug Administration/Center for Drug Evaluation and Research

ACE Inhibitors

"ACE" is an acronym for angiotensin-converting enzyme. Angiotensin is produced by your kidneys and is a chemical that causes blood vessels to constrict. The inhibitor helps the blood vessels to relax and open up. This makes it easier for the heart to pump blood through your body. They are prescribed for patients with high blood pressure or heart failure and after heart attacks. These are relatively new drugs and quite expensive. There is a newer group of drugs with similar characteristics, called angiotensin II receptor blockers.

Typical ACE inhibitors are Captopril, Enalapril, and Lisinopril.

HEART POINT

Aspirin is probably the best-selling drug in the world; about 50 billion aspirin tablets are consumed each year and 1 trillion since 1899. Hippocrates, around 400 B.C., discovered that chewing on willow bark could relieve pain and fever. The active ingredient in the willow is salicin, which was synthesized as acetylsalicylic acid by French chemists.

Aspirin and Anticoagulants

Aspirin is one of the most common and least expensive drugs for heart patients. Generally, it is not prescribed along with an anticoagulant. Aspirin is often given to those at high risk for heart disease and those who have recently had bypass surgery. Research suggests that it reduces the odds of new blockages forming in the newly grafted arteries. It and other anticoagulants are also prescribed after a stroke or heart attack. Doctors "prescribe" it to patients, even though it is available over-the-counter, to "thin" their blood and reduce the chance of blood clots forming. As it is taken daily, your doctor will determine the correct amount for you to take.

Coumadin (warfarin) is a frequently prescribed anticoagulant. All of the drugs in this category work to prevent blood clots that can lead to heart attack or stroke. They change or reduce the levels and interactions of proteins in blood that are involved in the clotting process, rather than actually "thinning" the blood.

Anticoagulant Problems

Aspirin is an irritant to your entire digestive tract and can cause bleeding. The amount and type of aspirin should be determined by your doctor. Taking it with food reduces the chance of irritation.

The major cause for concern for those taking anticoagulants is the possibility of "thinning the blood" too much. Over the long term, as many as 33 percent of those patients taking anticoagulants have some problem with serious bleeding. Older patients with arthritis need to be particularly careful. They often take anti-inflammatory drugs that are also irritating to the stomach. These include many of the nonsteroidal anti-inflammatory drugs (NSAIDs) that people are familiar with, such as ibuprofen (Advil and others), naproxen (Aleve and others), and other over-the-counter pain relievers such as acetaminophen (Tylenol). Combining the two types of drugs can be deadly. Over 10 percent of those patients hospitalized for bleeding peptic ulcer disease were combining NSAIDs and anticoagulants.

You also should be careful about maintaining the same daily consumption of foods high in vitamin K: broccoli, Brussels sprouts, spinach, other leafy green vegetables, and green tea. Vitamin K plays a significant part in the body's manufacture of clotting factors. So changing the amount of food you consume in this category will change the effectiveness of Coumadin.

Vitamin E, a frequently taken antioxidant, also acts to prevent blood clotting. Adding vitamin E could be dangerous if you are taking Coumadin. Ginkgo biloba also can add to the problem. Garlic supplements may present difficulties too, though the link is not as yet proven. Be aware of the potential problem and discuss it with your doctor.

The opposite effect may occur from the supplement coenzyme Q10 (ubiquinone). Many heart failure patients, along with those with other heart problems or gum disease, take this nutrient. Research suggests that it may interact with Coumadin and reduce its effectiveness.

Beta Blockers

Beta blockers work on the chemicals your nerve endings release. This reduces the heart rate and blood pressure. They are prescribed after a heart attack and for angina, arrhythmias, heart failure, and high blood pressure. Some patients taking beta blockers have problems with sleep disruption and fatigue. More serious potential side effects include breathing difficulties (call doctor

HEART POINT

WARNING: If you develop any new symptom after taking a new prescription drug, assume it is caused by the drug and call your doctor. If the symptom puts you in immediate danger, call 911.

immediately), worsening existing depression, and impotence in men. Diabetics taking beta blockers must watch for signs of low blood sugar. Sweating is one common sign. Typical beta blockers are propranolol (Inderal), metroprolol (Lopressor), nadolol (Corgard), and acebutolol (Sectral).

Calcium Channel Blockers

This group of drugs works by restricting calcium atoms from entering the muscle cells of the heart and blood vessels. Those muscles will not be able to contract as forcefully, and the arteries and heart relax somewhat. This helps dilate the coronary arteries, reduce heart rate, control arrhythmias, lower blood pressure, and prevent angina attacks.

Side effects can include constipation, headache, a rash, leg edema, and excessive reduction in blood pressure. Older adults have a higher risk of gastrointestinal bleeding. There may be some additional risk of cancer, though studies show very mixed results.

DARRELL'S STORY

"One of the 'small' side effects I experienced with calcium channel blockers was an increase in gum disease problems. After much discussion and continued monitoring, my health team, including me, has decided to stay with this class of drugs. I counteract the side effects by diligent gum care, three-times-per-year visits to the periodontist for scaling, and the addition of another drug, a low-dose antibiotic, to fight the gum disease. The chemistry experiment continues."

Typical calcium channel blockers are diltiazem (Cardizem), verapamil (Calan, Isoptin, Verelan), and amlodipine (Norvasc). Avoid drinking grapefruit juice and eating grapefruit when taking this class of drugs. In one study, combining this healthy juice plus the prescribed drug increased the drug's availability to the body by over 134 percent. This dangerous change in the patient's body produced flushing, headaches, and light-headedness.

Cholesterol Medications

There are a number of different types of cholesterol medications. Some primarily act to reduce LDL ("bad") cholesterol. Others types work to lower triglycerides or to raise HDL ("good") cholesterol.

Statins are the kind that have most been featured in the news recently. A recent study reported in the *New England Journal of Medicine* reported that patients taking simvastatin along with niacin had a lower risk of heart attack, an increase in HDL, and lower LDL. This combination may benefit patients with low HDL, one independent risk factor for heart disease. All of the statin drugs increase your body's ability to dispose of cholesterol. Niacin (nicotinic acid) limits the body's ability to produce more very low-density lipoprotein (VLDL) cholesterol. Gemfibrozil raises HDL cholesterol while reducing VLDL cholesterol and triglycerides. Side effects vary by specific drug, though many can cause stomach upset, nausea, headache, or blurred vision. Watch for and report any new muscle aches to your doctor. Most require monitoring of liver function that requires testing every few months.

Typical cholesterol drugs are gemfibrozil (Lopid), lovastatin (Mevacor), pravastatin (Pravachol), simvastatin (Zocor), and niacin (Niacels, Nicolar, and others).

HEART POINT

Heart patients should work to keep their LDL cholesterol under 100 and HDL over 40. Improve your lifestyle through diet and exercise as much as possible to minimize the necessity of drug use.

Digitalis

Digitalis, traditionally extracted from the plant foxglove, has a long history as an herbal medicine, though today's medicine is mostly produced synthetically. Doctors prescribe it to control certain types of arrhythmias and heart failure. There is some evidence that it is over-prescribed for heart failure. Your doctor will need to periodically monitor the levels of digitalis in the blood because of the risk of toxic effects. Be very careful about how you take digitalis. Follow all mixing instructions exactly. If you are using the liquid form, use only the special marked dropper for measuring. Monitor your pulse after taking the drug. If your pulse drops below sixty beats per minute, consult with your physician. There are many potential drug interactions that need to be discussed with your doctor. Typical digitalis drugs are digoxin (Lanoxin) and digitoxin (Crystodigin).

HEART POINT

Adding foods high in potassium, such as bananas and orange juice, may help balance shortages caused by some diuretics.

Diuretics

Diuretics work to remove water from your body, which in turn decreases blood pressure. They are among the most widely prescribed and least expensive classes of drugs available. They can be the starting point of treatment or used in combination with other drugs and are prescribed for heart failure and high blood pressure. Side effects can include an imbalance of potassium, calcium, or sodium, so those should be monitored regularly. Some diuretics raise glucose so diabetics should manage sugar levels carefully. When taking diuretics, avoid regular use of laxatives. It's best to take diuretics early in the day to help decrease urination at night. Typical diuretics are chlorothiazide (Diuril), hydrochlorothiazide (Esidrix, hydroDIURIL, and Oretic), and furosemide (Lasix).

Vasodilators

Several of the classes of drugs that we have already discussed can be considered vasodilators—medicine that dilates, or widens, the peripheral arteries in your body. ACE inhibitors, calcium channel blockers, and nitrates all work to reduce the work level of the heart through this process. Specifics are described in the respective sections.

Sexual Side Effects

Sex is an important part of life. Many drugs used for treating various heart conditions can cause sexual dysfunction. Effects vary by individual and dosages, but if you experience any problem, discuss it with your doctor. There are often alternative drug choices that can be tried instead of the problem drugs. Blood pressure drugs, including beta blockers, some diuretics, and others, can present major problems.

SURGICAL TREATMENTS FOR HEART DISEASE

AS VARIOUS FORMS of heart disease worsen and cause additional problems, doctors might recommend surgery. We describe some types of invasive procedures and surgery that are now regularly performed.

HEART POINT

WARNING: Impotence drugs, including Viagra, can be dangerous for individuals with heart problems and those taking heart medications—proceed with caution.

Impotence drugs, including Viagra, may interact with drugs given immediately after a heart attack. If you have taken one of these drugs and have a heart attack, inform emergency medical technicians and emergency room personnel.

Coronary Angioplasty

The surgeon makes an incision in your groin, then in your artery. He will insert a catheter—a long, thin, flexible tube—and thread it through your blood vessels to the heart. During the angiogram, he will inject a dye into your body so your coronary arteries can be viewed with X-rays. If the surgeon determines that there's a significant blockage that cuts off blood flow inside an artery, he may proceed with a coronary angioplasty (technically called a percutaneous transluminal coronary angioplasty, or PTCA).

The surgeon inserts a second, smaller catheter into the blocked area. That catheter has a tiny inflatable balloon at the tip. The surgeon inflates the balloon for 30 to 120 seconds and may need to repeat this several or many times until the balloon pushes the artery back open. Once the artery is open, the surgeon frequently inserts a stent into the area of the former blockage. A stent is a metal-mesh

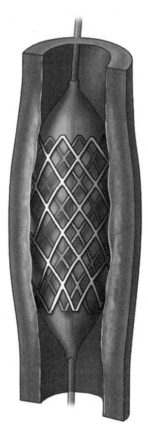

After the blockage has been opened, a stent is often placed inside the artery to help keep blood flowing. Copyright © 2002 Nucleus Communications, Inc. All rights reserved. www.nucleusinc.com

tube that looks a bit like a child's Chinese finger puzzle that springs open and holds the artery open after the surgery. The angioplasty, with a stent, is successful about 70 percent to 80 percent of the time. Several new techniques are being tested to reduce the failure rate, including using specially coated stents or inserting a small piece of radioactive material for a short time after the surgery. Both experiments are promising, though still experimental.

In some hospitals this is a multiday process, with the angiogram done the first day to determine your status, and the procedure to open the artery done on the second day. We think it's generally better to go to a hospital that does it during the same visit to the "cath lab." This minimizes time in the hospital and chances for complications.

DARRELL'S STORY

"I don't remember being afraid about my angioplasty. It seemed so routine, such an everyday procedure, yet fascinating. I was struck by all the personnel in an amazingly high-tech operating room. I was awake and watching the monitor. In a way, it is an out-of-body experience; it seems a bit like watching a health program on TV or being in the sick bay on the Starship *Enterprise*, except it's your body and not fiction. I remember the surge of warmth when the surgeon injected the contrast fluid through my body. Someone turned on the X-ray and my arteries appeared on the screen; they twitch, twist, turn, and bulge. I really couldn't sort out the good from the bad; I wanted to, but didn't really know what I was looking at. (I did get better at it with practice, unfortunately.) The surgeon told me that I had a blockage and that he would go out and tell my wife, Geri. He didn't tell me, but told her, that my left anterior descending artery was 100 percent closed and they would attempt to open it up. I believe that the risk of complications, heart attack, or stroke was much higher than with a lesser blockage. He explained to her that if they couldn't open the blockage I would have to have a bypass. The surgeon returned to the operating room and told me he was going forward. I suspect that that is when they increased the 'happy juice' in my system; I fell asleep. Looking back, I'm convinced that that was a conscious move on the surgical team's part to prepare me for the worst-case scenario. I woke a few minutes later and heard that my artery was now open. I felt better immediately—a combination of relief that it was over and the physical reality that blood was now flowing again.

"The worst part of the procedure was having my leg and groin area immobile for over six hours. I had a slight problem with bleeding from the incision and had to be in bed a bit longer than normal. As soon as that was resolved, I was up and out of bed. An aide wheeled me out of the hospital (hospital policy). At the front door, I got out of the wheelchair, started walking, and felt great, better than I had for months. I was a new man and free of heart disease—I thought. I walked up the hill to a restaurant for some real food. Leaving there, I wanted to take the subway home; Geri insisted on a cab. I had no recovery time. I returned to my normal life.

"I thought it was all over—someone sticks a tube in you, cleans you out, and you go back to eating cheeseburgers. Modern science had saved me—or so I thought. That was in March. A few months later, another surgeon opened a blockage within the stent, with a cutting device (called a 'roto-rooter') on the end of a catheter. In August, I had my third angioplasty with another stent. The surgeons warned me then that if I had more blockages, I would need a bypass. There was no real pain during my angioplasty, only some pressure when the balloons were inflated."

Bypass Surgery

A coronary artery bypass grafting operation (CABG, a "cabbage" to most people) is quite simple in principle. It's like adding new sections of pipe (arteries) around blocked areas to restore blood flow. In practice, this is a complex and difficult operation, even though there are about 600,000 performed each year.

You are given general anesthesia and are totally asleep during the procedure. The chest cavity is opened, and you are attached to the heart–lung machine. The heart–lung machine assumes the functions of both organs so the surgeon can work on a nonbeating heart. A leg vein or arm artery is harvested. One end is connected to the aorta close to the heart and the other end is connected farther down the coronary artery at a point past the blockage. A third possibility is using one or both of the internal mammary arteries. The surgeon removes the end downstream, which is on the inner chest wall. That is reconnected to the coronary artery at a point past the blockage. The mammary arteries may be totally removed and then reattached. All of the procedures redirect blood flow around the blocked area.

New Bypass Variations

Some patients may benefit from new types of bypass surgery. Minimally invasive bypass is less traumatic for the patient's body and speeds recovery. Surgery is done through a small incision rather than through the open chest (one area of potential complication). Beating heart surgery eliminates the need for the heart–lung machine. This avoids all of the machine risks and may be particularly suited to older patients. Working with a beating heart is one of the most challenging procedures. For all new procedures, it takes years for surgeons to develop the highest skill levels and for analyses to be done. Many of these procedures are available only for patients with one- and two-vessel disease.

Valve Replacement Surgery

Surgery to replace valves that are not functioning correctly begins like bypass surgery. You are under general anesthesia, the chest cavity is opened, and you are placed on the heart–lung machine. The bad valves are removed and replaced with valves made of a variety of materials. Recovery takes place over several months.

Pacemaker Installation

This is a "relatively minor" type of heart surgery, taking only about an hour and done under local anesthesia. Your chest is scrubbed and numbed, then opened.

Wires are placed into a vein and threaded to the right side of your heart. The doctor then tests the device to make sure the placement is optimized. The pulse generator is then implanted in a pocket beneath the skin.

Heart Transplant

As options for repair of the heart diminish, a heart transplant becomes a final possibility. In some cases the whole heart is removed and replaced with a donor heart. There are only a few thousand such transplants each year because of the difficulties of locating donor hearts. Some heart transplants are in fact only partial transplants, with the ventricles (the two main pumping chambers), valves, and parts of the atria (the two smaller chambers of the heart) removed from a donor heart and then attached onto the recipient's heart. Patients must take immunosuppressive drugs immediately after the operation and for the rest of their lives. More experimentation is being done with support pumps for individuals whose heart is failing, with promising initial results.

OTHER TREATMENTS

Enhanced External Counterpulsation (EECP)

A noninvasive treatment for angina that has shown positive results is EECP. New data was presented at the American Heart Association Scientific Sessions in November 2000. EECP is a mechanical treatment using cuffs (like blood pressure cuffs) around the patient's legs. The cuffs are inflated and deflated in sequence with the heartbeat. When the heartbeat ends, a computer signals inflation of the cuffs that pushes the blood in the legs upward toward the heart.

Treatments increase the blood flow to the coronary arteries, which get their blood flow in cycles after the heartbeat. The treatment increases blood flow to the heart.

Patients get five one-hour treatments each week for a seven-week period (thirty-five treatments in all). The treatments are effective in treating stable angina; they lessen lessons symptoms and improve exercise tolerance. Research suggests that this treatment works for up to five years. It may help other patients with angina. It is not suited for patients who have some types of valve disease, irregular heart rhythms, severe hypertension, significant blockages in leg arteries, blood clots in legs, or who have had a recent cardiac catheterization.

Some experts have suggested that this treatment is not widespread because of the lower financial return to cardiologists. The thirty-five sessions cost about $7,000 for thirty-five hours of work instead of about $18,000 for angioplasty or more than $40,000 for a CABG. The treatment is available only in about 200 centers in the United States. Medicare and many insurance companies have approved it for reimbursement. If your insurance company doesn't reimburse, you can appeal. In another trial, thallium stress testing showed that 75 percent of patients had improvements along with improved exercise tolerance. Some patients who are not suitable candidates for surgery may be able to use EECP.

Chelation

Chelation is a chemical process that removes unwanted substances from other liquids. For heart patients, the theory is that chelation with EDTA (ethylene-diamine-tetra-acetate) removes artery-clogging substances from our blood and arteries. A recent trial in Calgary, Canada, and reported in the January 23, 2002, issue of the *Journal of the American Medical Association,* showed that it offered no benefit to patients with coronary artery disease and stable angina. This was a controlled double-blind study with some of the patients with heart disease getting the chelation treatment and others a placebo. There was no improvement in the group who received chelation rather than the placebo. Almost 8 percent of those getting standard cardiac care also are doing chelation on the side, so a lot of money is being spent for a procedure that does not seem to have any benefit.

STAR POINT FIVE

Live Heart Smart

*"We study health, and we deliberate upon our meats and drink
and air and exercises, and we hew and we polish every stone that
goes to the building; and so our health is a long and regular work."*

—JOHN DONNE, *Devotions upon Emergent Occasions, Meditation 1* (1624)

IT'S NOT ALWAYS easy to do the right thing for our bodies and our health. Individuals often grasp at any excuse or lie to themselves in order to avoid doing what's best. Many of the people who have already had a heart attack don't change their habits or improve their lifestyle in any way. There are no simple, quick fixes for heart disease. Bypass surgery and angioplasties only provide relief from symptoms. They do not cure heart disease. Simply cutting back a little bit on fat and hitting the treadmill once in a while is not going to protect anyone from heart disease (though, every little bit does help). To prevent or reverse heart and cardiovascular disease the patient must use a multi-faceted approach. We have known that improving our heart-healthy behavior for each of the individual risk factors adds years to our lives. Now, we know from the Harvard Nurses' Health Study that eating a low-fat, high-fiber diet, combined with an active lifestyle, moderate drinking, and avoiding smoking can reduce your risk of stroke, heart disease, and congestive heart failure by an amazing 82 percent (four-fifths). Though the Harvard Nurses' Health Study looked mostly at women, the huge improvement in odds is likely to apply to women and men equally.

The single most important element in improving your odds in the fight against cardiovascular disease is you! If you make the choice, you can help your body fight this disease. There is no magic bullet; no pill, no machine, and no surgery that will make heart disease disappear. The "secret" is an improved lifestyle: combine an active lifestyle with cutting stress, eating a low-fat, high-fiber diet, moderate drinking, and no smoking. These choices can help patients work toward reversing heart disease, yet many doctors, and the American Heart Association, do not do enough to educate patients. This section of *Surviving with Heart* encourages you to take charge of your health, but you have to decide. This is the first step in your long-term survival and the major "secret" of surviving, reversing, and beating cardiovascular disease. We give you steps to improve your odds that include cutting stress, eating a low-fat, high-fiber diet, controlling blood pressure and blood sugar, exercising, and stopping smoking. We also emphasize the role of cardiac rehabilitation for those already diagnosed with a condition and those at high risk for heart disease.

> "There is no magic bullet; no pill, no machine, and no surgery that will make heart disease disappear. The "secret" is an improved lifestyle."

DARRELL'S STORY

"I know that living heart smart and staying healthy takes an unbelievable amount of time, but consider the alternative. I now know that my angioplasties and bypass surgery only relieved my symptoms and if I don't live right and prevent future blockages, I will be back in the hospital. Each surgery will be higher risk and I don't want that. I want to live! So, this is the plan I'm following to stay healthy and to survive."

CONTROL STRESS

"As a man thinketh in his heart, so is he."

—PROVERBS 23:7

THE OVERWHELMING, UGLY monster is *stress*. There are two constants in life. The first is change, and it causes the second—stress. We face potentially stressful things every day. Stress affects different people in different ways. Many experts consider stress a contributing factor to heart disease. But after the heart attack occurs and the damage is done, how can the patient and caregiver handle stress better? The key is purposefully handling it.

Stress is a killer. Research suggests that stress causes more and greater problems than anyone has previously realized. Estimates vary, but some authorities suggest that between 75 percent and 90 percent of all visits to doctors are complaints and diseases that are stress related. As many as 43 percent of the adult population suffer some negative health effects from stress. The American Psychological Association estimates that stress costs American industry over $300 billion, about $7,500 per employee. The Occupational Safety and Health Administration has declared stress an official hazard in the workplace. Your job, or the threat of losing a job, commuting, children, and aging parents all add stress to everyday life. Even happy events like holidays, birthdays, weddings, getting a new job, or moving into a new house are major stress-producing events. Anything that happens to you affects your life and stress levels.

HEART POINT

A man is thinking to himself, "It's 7:30, my wife is already waiting for me. We're going to be late for that dinner party." Then he yells at the driver in the car ahead of him. His breathing and blood pressure increase and his heart rate speeds up. His whole body tightens; the muscles in his arms, shoulders, and neck stiffen; he feels his face get warmer. His digestive system shuts down. He is now ready to fight the woolly mammoth.

Modern man has vestiges of protective mechanisms from our caveman ancestors. The so-called flight-or-fight response that was provoked within our ancestors' bodies with the threatening approach of the woolly mammoth, saber-toothed tiger, or other enemy is the same response we have to being cut off on the expressway, or when someone slips into the parking space we are waiting for, or in many other everyday situations. These responses create substantial chemical and physical changes in our bodies. What are short-term protective mechanisms become long-term disasters for our bodies. Chronic stress is a killer.

The Harmful Effects of Stress

"In the world ye shall have tribulation."
—JOHN 16:33

How does stress affect the body, and how harmful is it? There is a general feeling that stress is bad for us—we know it—even if we can't point to specific evidence. But there is evidence of what stress does to the body. That "flight-or-fight" response produces specific reactions. As we prepare to "do battle," our heart races into action and starts pumping more blood into our system, causing our blood pressure to soar. Our breathing keeps pace, increasing in speed to provide more oxygen for our tensing muscles. Sweat starts to flow out of every pore of our body.

Other changes occur that we can't feel. Our digestion slows, because the blood has been redirected to our muscles and our brain, where it's needed more. Chemicals, fats, and sugars pour into our blood. Hormones, including adrenaline, help prepare the body for physical action and cause blood to clot more readily. That's important during a battle with the saber-toothed tiger, much less so in a heated, verbal exchange with the boss. Those hormones also lead to higher acidity in the stomach. And perhaps worst of all, those hormones pouring into the bloodstream interfere with the immune system of the body and its ability to fight off disease.

Even if stress didn't have direct negative effects on the body, it can lead to negative behaviors, which do have disastrous consequences. It can lead to smoking, drinking, drug abuse, and overeating; all can destroy our bodies. We also know that stress can produce skin problems, including hives and eczema.

Symptoms of Stress

There are some obvious and other not-so-obvious signs that persons are suffering with stress. Physically they may be plagued with headaches, fatigue, muscle aches and pains, heart palpitations, and sweating. They may also suffer with frequent colds. Individuals may be mentally challenged with confusion, indecisiveness, less concentration and memory, or a loss of their sense of humor. Emotionally they face symptoms of nervousness, frustration, worry, fear, irritability, and anger. Their behavior may change too, including nervous habits such as foot tapping, nail biting, fidgeting, and pacing. They may act out by swearing, yelling, throwing things, or hitting, or by increasing their eating, drinking, and smoking.

HEART POINT

STRESS REDUCER: Take an anger management or stress reduction course; it could save or add years to your life.

Stress and Heart Disease

While there is no definitive study that proves that stress causes heart disease and premature death, there is a great deal of circumstantial evidence. We know that the serum level of the amino acid homocysteine, a risk factor for coronary artery disease, increases during stress. An article in the journal *Circulation,* in May 2000, concludes that people who are quick to anger have an increased risk of heart disease. Those individuals who have an outburst of anger are twice as likely to have a heart attack in the few hours following the episode as others. James Blumenthal and other researchers at Duke University showed participants who were trying to solve difficult math problems experienced stress that constricted the coronary arteries. A number of studies have shown that people who have gone through major life changes (a job loss, a divorce or loss of spouse or close relative, or moving to a new location) are more likely to die younger than those who haven't. Dr. Dean Ornish has shown in his research and books that many individuals can reverse coronary artery disease by faithfully following a program of stress reduction, exercise, and a low-fat diet. One group of patients with coronary artery disease significantly reduced their risk of heart attacks by following a program of smoking cessation, weight loss, and control of lipids combined with a formal stress management program.

Type A Behavior

> *"But he that hides a dark soul and foul thoughts*
> *Benighted walks under the mid-day Sun:*
> *Himself is his own dungeon."*
>
> —JOHN MILTON, *Comus* (1637)

Most people have heard about Type A behaviors. Drs. Meyer Friedman and Ray Rosenman led the way in the 1950s studying this coronary-prone behavior pattern. They started out to study the relationship of stress to heart disease and discovered specific behavior traits that seemed to relate to a high level of heart disease. These Type A men seem to aggressively fight to achieve more in less time than other men do. They are almost obsessive about it. They often have machine-gun speech patterns, trying to quickly get to the end of sentences or interrupt others and finish their sentences. They are impatient with others and attempt to do two or more things at the same time. They think about business problems during leisure activities, they read and eat at the same time, and they can rarely relax, even on vacation. They are aggressive, impatient, and very competitive.

In this constant battle, the "flight-or-fight" response is almost continually triggered, with disastrous consequences. The hormones adrenaline and cortisol pump into the bloodstream along with cholesterol and fat. This increases clotting in the blood and makes it difficult for the body to rid the bloodstream of cholesterol. Of 3,000 healthy men that the doctors interviewed for the Western Collaborative Group Study, within eight and one-half years, the half classified as Type A had twice the incidence of coronary heart disease as the other half. Type A's also are more likely to have high blood pressure and diabetes.

Changing Type A Behaviors

> *"We boil at different degrees."*
>
> —RALPH WALDO EMERSON, *Society and Solitude* (1870)

There is controversy about whether a true Type A personality exists, but we know that Type A behaviors do. The behaviors need to be changed. It is difficult but not impossible to change Type A behaviors. Our society values and rewards some of those behaviors. We also know that those behaviors add a significant risk of heart disease and heart attack to our lives. Several studies have been done that show you can modify the behaviors and decrease the risk of a heart attack. The patients are given intensive behavioral training with the objectives of getting them to slow down, to be less goal oriented, and to enjoy the process of tasks and life. They are also taught to be more patient and to improve their outlook to become more positive. One of the keys to success is to show Type A's that their lifestyle is actually inefficient and that they will actually accomplish more by learning to slow down and enjoy life and appreciate each step needed to complete a task.

Reducing Stress in Our Lives

The response of the man mentioned earlier who is late and fighting traffic was not caused by the driver in front of him, but by not planning well. We often can avoid stress, or minimize it, by simply allowing a few extra minutes in our daily schedules, simply being more realistic. By allowing extra time for heavy traffic, we will not be as stressed. What are some of the other strategies to reduce stress in our lives? Some of the strategies we discuss include: meditation; yoga; laughter; deep breathing; assertiveness; a positive attitude; a strong support network of family, friends, and caregivers; exercise; acceptance; avoidance; and altering. What follows is only an introduction to some of the methods of reducing stress. The most important thing is learning to recognize the stress in your life, then working to avoid chronic stress. You cannot eliminate stress from your life, but you can learn to control it. Following are some approaches to controlling stress in your lives.

Writing About Stress

Take twenty minutes and write out the most stressful event of your life. Continue writing for the full twenty minutes—don't cheat. Do this for three straight days. You can write about the same stressful event or day at each session or write about another stress-laden example (who doesn't have more than one?). This exercise duplicates an actual medical research experiment. A number of asthma sufferers were split into two groups; one group wrote about their

> "You cannot eliminate stress from your life, but you can learn to control it."

stressful days and the control group wrote about neutral topics. Four months later, researchers evaluated the health of both groups. Over 47 percent of the group that wrote about stressful events showed clinically significant improvement in their health as opposed to only 24 percent of the control group showing improvement.

Exercise

A complete section later in this chapter deals with all of the heart-healthy benefits of exercise. Here we simply look at exercise as a stress reducer. Think of how the body becomes aroused into a high-energy state when it prepares to "do battle" with the saber-toothed tiger or a difficult person. We need a relief valve to dissipate that excess energy before it can do harm. If conditions allow it, going for a fast walk will immediately help your body and mind. That doesn't duplicate the battle to the death with the enemy but does use up that energy. Consider exercise a modern equivalent. The exercise seems to use up the hormones and other chemicals that are dumped into our blood.

HEART POINT

STRESS REDUCER: Do some gardening; being outside and working with plants are good ways to reduce stress.

Once they are used up, they cannot attack the blood vessels, heart, and immune system.

Besides removing chemicals that produce negative actions and results, exercise stimulates the brain and releases endorphins into our bodies. Endorphins produce positive and happy feelings. When you finish exercising, you can feel exhausted, but you feel good, much calmer, and more relaxed than before.

A regular exercise program helps dissipate the ongoing buildup of chronic stress. Many, if not most, people are under stress on a constant basis. Life is full of stresses. It makes sense to exercise regularly to have a consistent outlet for the stress. It is best to do something at least three times a week for a minimum of thirty minutes each session. More frequent exercise and exercise of longer duration are even better.

Choose an activity that you like. We are much more likely to stay with a program if we enjoy what we are doing. It doesn't matter whether you walk, jog, swim, ski, dance, take aerobics classes, or use some other form of exercise. In many ways, walking is an ideal pursuit. It requires no special equipment, other than a good pair of walking shoes, and a bit of time.

HEART POINT

STRESS REDUCER: Forgive people; we do not live in a perfect world. Accept the fact that you and others make mistakes, forgive them and yourself, and move on. You will be much happier.

DARRELL'S STORY

"I felt pressure and stress at several points during the writing of this book. Ironically, one moment occurred during the writing of the section on stress. I think the looming deadline, extended twice already, was hanging over my head; it seemed to be closing in on me. I was running out of time; printing schedules, catalogs, and editing deadlines were set. I became more aware of my reactions; I was irritable and having trouble sleeping. That awareness made me analyze my situation. First, I thought what is the worst thing that could happen if I did not make the book deadline? Well, the book would be delayed, printed, and sold in the next season. My editor would get over it. Next, I started exercising a bit more. I had let my regular exercise slip in order to have more time for writing. It was time to get back on track and do my four-mile walk each day. Then I made a new effort to eat well, rather than just grab something on the run. All of these things improved my attitude, I felt better, and I was even able to write more. And as I review this a few days prior to the final deadline, I'm still not sure if we will make it. I do care and am working hard, but I'm not letting it make me sick. My health is more important than this book."

Exercise also gives you a sense of control over your body and life. Much stress is produced because of your feeling of lack of control over your life and low self-esteem. By starting to exercise and staying with it, you do have more control and start to improve your overall perception of your life and body.

Meditation and Relaxation Techniques

In the 1960s, the United States experienced many things, including the British invasion in music, hippies, and Transcendental Meditation™. Many people questioned the worth of each of those. Over decades, research has shown the worth of meditation, though the other two continue to be debated. Dr. Herbert Benson, in his book *The Relaxation Response,* showed how meditation helps lower blood pressure and deal with stress. It can produce physiologic changes in our bodies that reverse those of a body under stress. Our heart rate and breathing slow, tense muscles relax, and blood pressure drops.

While our body's reaction to stress is automatic, meditation must be sought out consciously. The best way to learn is through a course or some formal training seminar, though you can learn the basics from books and tapes. Meditation is a process rather than a goal, and you should focus on the moment rather than the fact that meditation is good for you and may help you live longer. The focus is generally your breathing or a sound such as "ahhhh," "ohhhhh," or "ohm." If your mind wanders, as it probably will, firmly, yet gently, return to your breathing or the sound.

HEART POINT

SIMPLE MEDITATION: Find a quiet spot where you can avoid moving for about twenty minutes. Sit or lie on the floor and keep your back straight, but not stiff. Focus on your breathing, counting each breath. Keep your breathing slow, yet natural, and count up to ten, then start over.

Deep Breathing

Many relaxation techniques use some form of deep breathing. It's a good first step and can be combined with other activities. It is an antidote to stress, as stress causes us to breathe in shallow breaths. Start with good posture, either standing or sitting, and place your hands on your stomach. Inhale slowly and deeply through your nose and allow your stomach to expand. Your hands will feel your stomach expand as you breathe in as much as you can. Hold your breath several seconds before exhaling.

Reverse the process and exhale through your mouth. Purse your lips, like you are going to whistle. This slows the process, which is the point. You will feel your stomach deflate. This also expands the diaphragm. Keep exhaling until your lungs feel empty, then start the process over again. When you do this exercise for the first time, aim to go through about four complete inhalation–exhalation cycles in order to get the full benefit.

HEART POINT

STRESS REDUCER: Have fresh flowers where you work and live.

Visualization

When you feel stressed, take a trip via your mind—visualize a safe, comforting, relaxing, and beautiful place. Go beyond simply thinking about the place, actually put yourself there. Start to be aware of the sounds, the smells, and the temperature. This visualization will transport you to a place of tranquility.

DARRELL'S STORY

"My favorite visualization is a place on a tropical island. It may be the Caribbean, Hawaii, or Fiji, depending on the day. I am lying in a large, rope hammock strung between two palm trees swaying in the wind. The palm fronds rustle as the warm breeze blows. I sway a little as I roll a little onto my side to look at a three-masted sailboat on the deep blue water. The warm breeze carries the scent of salt air and tropical flowers over me. I hear waves crashing and seabirds splashing into the water fishing for their lunch; occasionally, I hear steel drums or Jimmy Buffett singing. Whenever I need it, the visualization transports me into the land of calm."

Other Relaxation Techniques

Most other relaxation techniques need you to "clear your mind." Biofeedback, done with the help of a professional, teaches you to monitor your reaction to stress. A simple set of stretching exercises will help relieve muscle tension that often accompanies stress. There are also several "progressive" techniques, which guide you to relax specific body parts or muscle groups. Autogenics uses "mind over matter" by having you focus on a specific body part—your right arm, for instance—thinking that it is warm and heavy. Once it "feels" that way, move progressively through the rest of the body. Progressive muscle relaxation is similar, though you progressively tense, then release, specific muscle groups.

Pets

Millions of Americans love their pets, but most don't realize how healthful they are. Dogs and cats seem to lower blood pressure and cholesterol. Pet owners have a higher chance of surviving a heart attack than nonowners. Two studies looked at patients about to have a physical exam from a doctor. A dog was put into the exam room with children, and dogs and

---

HEART POINT

STRESS REDUCER: Fix or replace small things that do not work and are a constant aggravation. These may include a dripping faucet, a car rattle, or malfunctioning weedwhacker, can opener, or windshield wipers.

cats were used similarly for a group of stockbrokers. The distress, heart rate, and blood pressure of the patients was lower after the dogs and cats were introduced. And who can deny the simple pleasures of patting a dog sitting next to you or stroking a purring cat on your lap. Another recent study published in the October 2001 issue of the journal *Hypertension* showed pet owners had less of an increase in heart rate and blood pressure in stressful situations than did a control group of people without pets.

Learning to Say "No"

Many people struggling with stress simply take on too many responsibilities. You know the problem. You are striving hard to finish a major project in the office and already putting in extra hours, yet agree to join the coop board in your building, coach the Little League team, or raise money for your church. Most people don't want to disappoint others or to be seen as lazy or not helpful. Learn to say "yes" to only those activities that will bring you pleasure or ones that you believe are important. Once you are a heart patient, that provides the perfect solution. When someone asks you to do one more job you really don't have time for, just say, "My cardiologist told me not to take on any new responsibilities." As an alternative, say, "I just don't believe I have enough time to do the project justice."

DARRELL'S STORY

"After my first angioplasty, my cardiologist suggested I reduce stress in my life. At the time, I was president of the Long Island Horticultural Society, handling many committees myself, along with being on a number of other nonprofit boards of directors. I resigned all of the boards except LIHS and recruited volunteers to take on some of the other jobs I had been doing. I was set to announce these changes at the next board meeting. I called the meeting to order and said I had a few announcements. I informed everyone of my hospitalization and angioplasty and said, 'My cardiologist told me to reduce my stress.' The board broke into laughter, realizing that continuing as president was not the way to do that."

Altering

Another way of dealing with stress is to alter the situation. This is easiest to do with our physical environment. Things that might cause stress but are fairly easy to alter include a dripping faucet, an uncomfortable chair to work in, or bad lighting. With a little effort and investment we can remove those sources of stress.

Avoidance

Our society generally has a bad feeling about people who avoid things. "Be a man, face up to your problem." While it's true that many problems need to be faced and worked on with a hope of solving them, many stress-producing situations are best handled by avoiding them. Why not avoid the boss when she is unhappy and "looking for a fight"? Don't continue to drive a particular route to work if it is always crowded or loaded with aggressive drivers. Better yet, don't drive to work if there is an alternative such as public transportation or a car pool available. Also, don't spend time with negative people or those who are going to add stress to your life; avoid them and you will eliminate some stress from your life.

HEART POINT

STRESS REDUCER: Preset your morning by laying out your clothes, setting the breakfast table, fixing lunch, and cooking your steel-cut oats (whole oats cut into a few pieces that take twenty to thirty minutes to cook) the night before.

Acceptance

Sometimes you just can't avoid or alter a situation to make it less stressful. You are stuck; what do you do then? It's best to find a way to accept the situation. Let's say you are stuck in traffic and you realize you will be late for a meeting or a dinner party. There are no alternative routes and nothing you can do to change your circumstances. Yelling and screaming at other drivers or inside the car isn't going to help in any way. Learn to accept things as they are, saying to yourself, "Those are the breaks." Turn on some soothing music on the car radio or listen to the CD you haven't been able to and finish your drive to your destination.

HEART POINT

STRESS REDUCER: Be prepared for delays and carry a paperback book to read in lines at the motor vehicle bureau or post office.

Learned Optimism

Being naturally optimistic or learning to be optimistic can protect you from stress and make you happier. Martin Seligman describes the optimistic "explanatory style" in his book *Learned Optimism.* Those who live that way view problems and troubles as short term rather than permanent. Confronted by a problem, such as heart disease, an optimist considers it a challenge and something to work harder at. The pessimist assumes it is a failure. Seligman suggests that there is evidence that optimists may live longer and are certainly healthier. We all have life challenges and setbacks; optimists simply handle them better. Pessimists can learn to change their response to life's stresses.

Massage

Massage seems like a pleasant indulgence, yet it has been shown to reduce stress. Even scientists don't know why it works, but it does. It certainly is a very nice form of relaxation. Studies have shown health benefits for men with HIV, whose immune system responses improved, and a study showed that a massage proved helpful to a group of medical workers, who achieved better results on timed math tests than a group of other workers who didn't get a massage.

HEART POINT

STRESS REDUCER: Do something nice for someone every day. Like the bumper sticker says, "Practice random acts of kindness!"

Laughter

We all like to laugh, and we do feel better afterward. Laughter stimulates physical changes in the body. Information from the Mayo Clinic suggests that laughter may reduce stress hormone levels, boost your immune system, ease pain, and relax your body. Norman Cousins started the trend of research into the value of humor after he was diagnosed with cancer, with little chance of recovery. After watching funny videos for eight days, his pain decreased and he was able to return to work. He tells his story in his book *Anatomy of an Illness.* Although researchers don't know why laughter works, they theorize that it releases endorphins, much like exercise does.

Even the anticipation of laughter has a positive effect. In a new study presented at the Society for Neuroscience meeting in November of 2001, Dr. Lee Berk described how a group of men, evaluated for signs of stress, was told they would get to watch a funny video in three days. Each man's mood improved progressively, even before seeing the video. Depression dropped 51 percent and anger dropped 19 percent two days before watching the video. After watching the video, anger and depression dropped 98 percent and tension 61 percent, with vigor increasing 37 percent. Humor, even just the anticipation of something funny, seems very positive for all of us.

Caregiver Stress

As a caregiver you have a choice as to how you deal with stress. Even if you are not aware of it, you could be using stress to gain control or get attention. Stress is habit-forming. It is easy to become used to complaining about your situation and finding things to be afraid of and stressed about. Some people who like being the center of attention find it difficult to have all the attention centered on their patient. They use stress as an excuse to lose control and get others to notice them. Caregivers who do not take time for themselves will begin to resent the time they focus on their patient's condition. Avoid using stress to get your needs met. It's a dead-end cycle. You get stressed, you get others and the patient more stressed, and you do physical and emotional damage to everyone.

ELLEN'S STORY

"I have a close friend who is a heart patient and a diabetic. Every time I talk with him, I will ask what his blood sugar was that morning or if he got to exercise. When he is feeling stressed or his schedule gets too busy, I try to casually talk about slowing down. It keeps the pressure on me to model a heart-smart lifestyle in front of him."

The Feeling Factor

In the first few weeks of your patient's recovery phase, you may hesitate to share your feelings for fear you will cause stress. It's during the recovery period that you need to find a trusted friend or counselor to talk with and vent your feelings. If you make sure you are working through feelings, then you will not be in danger of future emotional explosions that come from bottling up your emotions. You will be able to express your feelings to your patient and stay in control of yourself and your reactions.

In her book *Heartmates: A Guide for the Spouse and Family of the Heart Patient*, Rhoda Levin suggests taking three minutes every day just for sharing feelings. No response or answer is required. It is simply a time when you and your patient share with each other.

Sometimes, sitting down and talking about changes in diet and exercise is much less difficult than talking about feelings. But keeping your feelings bottled up and not sharing them in a conversational manner with your patient will cause you to blow up at some point in the future or to increase your risk of a heart attack because you did not practice stress reduction. If you find yourself eating more, check your stress level. Monitor feelings so you do not harm your body physically or emotionally or harm the relationship you have with your patient.

Face Fear

FRANK'S STORY
(caregiver, 54)

"When Alex had his heart attack, I didn't know what to do. About a week later I was angry at Alex, angry and afraid that he would leave me in some way. I had never thought about that before. I had taken things for granted and assumed he would always be there. We talked about it. We know each other very well and can work through problems quickly without a lot of words. We have been together twenty-nine years. Ultimately, the heart attack reminded us what we do have. It strengthened the relationship and what we mean to each other."

Fear is usually the first and most common feeling caregivers experience when their patients are diagnosed with some kind of heart problem. These feelings are completely normal and understandable, but giving in to constant fear drains them of needed emotional and physical energy. What kind of fears do most caregivers face?

HEART POINT

Constantly keep a check on why you are overeating. Hunger is rarely the culprit. For most people, anger, stress, frustration, loneliness, or boredom make up the real list of motivators. We use food to comfort us and distract us.

♦ **Fear of death**

Once you have faced a heart emergency, it is natural to fear another one. The realistic fact is that you probably will face another one. Heart disease requires a lifelong battle. Reading this Star Point helps you understand that it is possible to reverse the effects of heart disease only if the patient is willing to make critical life changes in how he or she eats, exercises, and reduces stress. Surgery and medication alone will not prevent another emergency.

Caregivers have acknowledged staying awake to listen to their patient breathe at night. Asking the doctor about any fearful areas will help you. Remember: *Information is powerful.* You can encourage your patient to commit to a healthier lifestyle, but you cannot control his breathing in the middle of the night. Don't waste your energy on things you can't change. It is easy for caregivers to imagine a multitude of exaggerated fears.

Giving in to fear can cause you to try and take too much control and act in an overly responsible way. Writing down your own feelings and journaling the health and feelings of your patient will keep you from calling the doctor every time your patient falls asleep earlier than usual or feels bad.

Talk to your patient about your fear. Set up a check-in system that lets you know where he or she is most of the time. Get a cellular phone so that you know your patient can call you if there is an emergency.

♦ Fear of abandonment

Caregivers not only fear for the loss of their patients but fear they will be left alone as a result. Enlarging your support systems will help you feel more stable. Make sure you know whom you can call with any kind of emergency or question—from medical to financial. (See Star Point Six for information on building a good support system.) If you allow yourself to focus on the fear of abandonment, you will soon begin to feel anger toward your patient. You will focus on your fear of the future and not find peace in enjoying every day. Your patient is alive, you are alive. Take the second chance and make the most of every day.

> "You didn't cause your patient's heart disease and you can't cure it."

LOU'S STORY
(caregiver, 56)

"I was devastated when my wife was diagnosed with heart disease and then had bypass surgery. I was so afraid she would die. The most frustrating thing was that I couldn't make it better for her. I couldn't 'fix it.' Men are supposed to do that. My brother finally talked point blank to me and said that if Sharon was going to die, I could not stop it. But if she was going to live, I could live with her. That was hard to hear, but it made me see what I had been doing. I was so afraid of her dying that I wasn't enjoying living with her."

♦ Fear of resuming sex

Caregivers fear the patient resuming normal activities. At the top of the list for many cardiac spouses is sexual activity. Just like any other physical activity, sex should be resumed gradually during the patient's recovery period. Waiting four to six weeks after surgery is recommended in order to give the incision time to heal. However, doctors suggest that snuggling is good from the beginning. Foreplay and mutual pleasuring is probably okay after two to three weeks. A couple may need to wait six weeks to participate in intercourse. Talk to your doctor, and let how the patient feels be your guide. Remember that sex takes about the same amount of energy as walking up a couple flights of stairs.

In her book *Heart Bypass: What Every Patient Must Know,* Gloria Hochman tells a story about a woman in her fifties who had been remarried for three months when she found out she had to have bypass surgery. Her first question to the doctor was about her survival chances and her second question was about sex. Most patients are concerned about sexual activity after surgery or a heart attack. When your patient feels comfortable about having sex again, you should too. Talk about it together. Ask the doctor about it together. If it's important to you, it's worth asking about.

Be aware that the depression many patients suffer after a heart attack or surgery can temporarily diminish sexual desires. This chapter offers information on combating impotency caused by medications.

Allow Anger

Caregivers are seldom prepared for their angry feelings. Their patient is confined to a hospital bed or recovering at home and the feelings start to creep in with no advance warning. Caregivers' anger takes on different forms.

DOROTHY'S STORY
(caregiver, 75)

"I dealt with my husband's heart condition for two years prior to his bypass surgery. I watched his energy level dwindle and his mental abilities decrease. I acted as the hostess for all the friends who came to offer support during the surgery. I barely left the hospital. In looking back, I guess

I calmed my fears by staying in control of everything. When he came home from the hospital I tended to get angry if he didn't listen to me or if he overdid it."

As caregivers, you can feel anger at your patients for getting heart disease and thinking they may leave you, at yourself for not seeing the symptoms, at the doctor, the hospital, or even at God. One caregiver said that she felt anger at her mother-in-law for not teaching her son better eating habits!

ELLEN'S STORY

"I was born and raised in the Deep South. I would have to get angry at generations of accomplished cooks and their unhealthy meals! You were not a good mom in the South if your children didn't clean their plates and eat all their fried chicken, creamed potatoes drenched in gravy, or their black-eyed peas flavored with hefty spoonfuls of bacon grease. But now my mother and I know better. We know what is healthy to cook and eat."

Fear can mount up and come out as anger, but much of the time it is caused by stress and frustration. The key is avoiding as much stress as possible so that you can keep angry feelings in check. If you are having trouble with anger, evaluate the following:

- Are you getting enough rest?
- Are you taking breaks and finding outlets that provide relaxation?
- Are you finding it difficult to get everything done?
- Are you having trouble focusing?
- What triggers an angry outburst from you?
- Are you communicating regularly and honestly with your patient?
- Do you have someone to talk with and share your feelings with on a regular basis?
- Do you practice techniques to help you stay calm?
- When you feel angry, what do you do?
- Are you getting enough exercise?

Understanding where your anger comes from, what triggers the feelings, and evaluating if you are taking good care of yourself will be of considerable help in overcoming the angry feelings. Excellent steps to stress reduction are provided in previous sections of this chapter.

Get Rid of Guilt

Guilt is often expressed through other emotions, such as anger. It can stifle positive communication and hinder the patient and caregiver from making progress in ongoing lifestyle management. There are two kinds of guilt that we feel. "Good guilt" is what some people call our conscience. It motivates us to make positive changes. For example, if you are eating ice cream in front of your heart patient and you feel bad about it, guess what? You should! Good guilt causes us to stop or start doing something that will make a difference. "Bad guilt" is the guilt we either "dump" on ourselves or allow others to "dump" on us. Bad guilt says we are not good enough. It affects our self-esteem, which either causes us to shut down or to strike out against someone else to make ourselves feel better. Bad guilt is feeling like you caused your patient's heart attack because you didn't cook healthy meals. Yes, you should have been eating healthier, but what your patient eats is ultimately his or her decision. You didn't cause your patient's heart disease and you can't cure it.

Make the personal lifestyle changes you need to make, make peace with anyone you need to, encourage your patient, and get on with life. Bad guilt is habit-forming. Get over it!

MARGIE'S STORY
(caregiver, 51)

"Every time someone talked about my mom's condition, I felt guilty. Somehow I felt responsible. If I had kept my dad from dying or gone to check on my mother more or made her eat better, she would not have gotten sick. By the time I got straightened out, I was so stressed out that my blood pressure was sky high."

Combat Confusion

DENISE'S STORY
(caregiver, 41)

"When my sister had her heart attack and then surgery, we were all at the hospital for two weeks. I was trying to work and take care of her teenage kids and my own kids. Even when she came home from the hospital, I took time off from work to stay with her. But after a couple of weeks of all the running back and forth, I had trouble just remembering what day it was."

Who wouldn't be confused? With every emotion under attack, a scary new world of medical information to absorb, and the concern over your loved one, caregiver confusion is absolutely normal and expected. However, confusion keeps you feeling overwhelmed and stops you from sorting out reality and details. Edward Charlesworth and Ronald Nathan warn against "awfulizing" in their book *Stress Management: A Comprehensive Guide to Your Well-Being.* We tend to think that it is awful if we can't manage things and keep everything going. The authors say that it is unfortunate if you can't manage, but it is not awful! Reserve awfulizing for traumatic events.

We both know how easy it is to get overwhelmed with all the demands of life in addition to dealing with heart disease. Try our four-step plan at any time during your caregiving journey to help you gain a realistic view of your situation.

Four Steps to Help You De-Awfulize
1. Prioritize
We are both "list" people. We make a "to-do list" every day. When you are under pressure emotionally and physically, your mental faculties need some help. Use the night before to think through what must be done the next day. Always ask the question, "Is this really necessary?" Many times we assume we have to do something because that is how we have been

doing it for some time. But in a crisis situation or an ongoing caregiving situation, you must constantly evaluate if something is really important. List only the important tasks that you can realistically accomplish.

2. Delegate

There will be times when getting the realistic task completed in one day takes the help of others. Let other people

> "Let other people help."

help. Ask others to help. Thinking that you are in charge of everything, every day, will kill you. If that is your tendency, you will act overly responsible. Be careful that you are not controlling tasks to fulfill your own needs, rather than focus on the patient.

Make a list of anyone who offers to help and add it to your list of family and friends who you know you can count on. Even if you add only one more person to your list, in addition to yourself, ask him or her to do some things. Look ahead and find a regular task that has to be done every week and ask someone to do it for you until your life calms down.

If you have problems with asking for help, go ahead and think about what kind of "thank-you" response you will give to those who help you. A note or card is always appreciated. Ask them over for dinner after your patient is feeling better. A "thank-you" gesture is appreciated at any time. Even if you don't get to respond to people for several months, it's okay.

3. Consult

Confusion can easily become habit-forming. After all, it is easier to stay confused than to find a way to combat it. But an easy way to reduce stress is to ask questions and get answers. Ask the doctor, ask the pharmacist, ask your neighbor who is a nurse, ask a friend at church or work. In Star Point Six we encourage you and your patient to embrace support. As you read that Star Point, think about enlarging your support list to include people who will answer your questions in any area. Write down numbers and addresses or keep them in a computer file. Make them easily accessible so you can get assistance as quickly as possible when you need information.

4. Simplify

Now's your opportunity. If you ever needed a reason to simplify your life, you have one now!

MARLA'S STORY
(caregiver, 42)

"When my mom got sick, I had to go see her all the time and stay and help and leave my own family. I finally got so stressed that I just started getting rid of everything that wasn't helping me out. I thought about giving away my kids and husband, but they talked me out of it! I started cooking meals that took less preparation, and we took a look at how busy all of us were each week and what we could cut out. We narrowed the kids' activities to one thing at a time. My daughter was taking gymnastics, piano, and wanted to play soccer. I talked to her and suggested she try one activity at a time and really focus on it to see if she liked it or not. There were some things we stopped doing that I miss, but I don't miss the stress."

It is time to look at the things that are really important to you and your family. Caring about a family member or loved one who has heart disease requires a lot of energy for a long time. What can you do to make your life easier? Giving up some activities and simplifying your lifestyle will reduce the stress in your life.

More Stress Reduction Ideas

Successful stress reduction is a necessary part of a healthy lifestyle. Other elements of that lifestyle help to further reduce stress. Good nutrition provides the quality "fuel" you need to maintain energy while avoiding the empty calories of junk food. Limiting or cutting out caffeine cuts out a stress-producing drug. Cut back your intake over a period of time to avoid withdrawal headaches.

Get enough sleep. Most people require from seven to eight hours sleep per night to actually awaken fully refreshed and able to handle the rigors of the days. Less will leave you tired and unable to cope with stressful situations. And remember to take time for yourself. Taking time for leisure activities and vacation is not only nice, but is a necessity. As stress builds we become fatigued and need the renewal from leisure activities.

EAT TO LIVE

HOW MANY PEOPLE do you know who say, "I've been on twenty-five different diets and I've lost 500 pounds. Yes, I lost 20 pounds on each one of them. Now, why am I 25 pounds heavier than when I started?"

Americans get fatter every year; much of our population is overweight or obese. Fat is everywhere we look: fast food, bacon cheese-burgers, French fries, ice cream, and donuts. The franchise outlets beckon us with give-aways, celebrities, and toys for the kids. Portions expand exponentially from regular to large to double to "bigger" and finally to the extra-biggie-jumbo-triple cheeseburger with three-quarters of a pound of high-fat ground beef with a quarter-pound of cheese and a bucket of French fries! Child-size portions are now larger than the adult-size portions that were originally served when the fast food chains first opened. The American diet is deadly. It is killing us. Heart disease is pervasive only in countries where the diet is high in fat and cholesterol. The few countries of the world with an even higher death rate from heart disease than ours have a diet that is even higher in fat and cholesterol than ours. What we eat along with the amount of exercise we do are major determining factors for our total weight and risk for heart disease. (Exercise is discussed in a separate section of this Star Point.)

HEART POINT

STRESS REDUCER: Eliminate caffeine in your diet. Try replacing it with herbal or green teas.

What's So Bad About Being Overweight?

The National Institute of Diabetes and Digestive and Kidney Diseases (NIDD-KD) is the part of the National Institutes of Health (NIH) that has the main responsibility for obesity- and nutrition-oriented research. NIDDKD points out that being overweight or obese are known risk factors for the following: diabetes, heart disease, stroke, hypertension, gallbladder disease, osteoarthritis, sleep apnea and other breathing problems, and some forms of cancer (uterine, breast, colorectal, kidney, and gallbladder). Obesity is also associated with high blood cholesterol, pregnancy complications, menstrual irregularities, and psychological disorders such as depression and adds risk to any surgical procedure.

> "Obesity causes over 280,000 adult deaths each year in the United States."

A recent survey detailed in the journal *Public Health* showed that obesity has more impact on our health than smoking, a known killer, and problem drinking. About 36 percent of those in the study were overweight, 23 percent obese, 19 percent daily smokers, and 6 percent heavy drinkers.

How Fat Are We?

The levels of obesity in the United States and much of the Western world are growing at epidemic proportions. Newspaper and magazine articles describe the ever-increasing numbers of men, women, and children who are fat. Between 1960 and 1994 the prevalence of overweight and obese individuals (BMI of 25 and higher) increased from 45.0 percent to 55.1 percent of the adult population of the United States. It is worse in minority populations over the age of twenty, with 65.8 percent of Black women, 65.9 percent of Mexican American women, 56.5 percent of Black men, and 63.9 percent of Mexican American men overweight or obese. Over $51.6 billion (1995), 5.7 percent of all U.S. health expenditures, are directly attributable to overweight and obesity. Obesity causes over 280,000 adult deaths each year in the United States.

What Is BMI (Body Mass Index)?

The relatively new measurement of choice for obesity and weight is the Body Mass Index (BMI). It is a calculated number based on weight and height. It's

BODY MASS INDEX TABLE

To use the table, find the appropriate height in the left-hand column labeled Height. Move across to a given weight. The number at the top of the column is the BMI at that height and weight. Pounds have been rounded off.

BMI	19	20	21	22	23	24	25	26	27	28	29	30	31	32	33	34	35
Height (inches)	**Body Weight** (pounds)																
58	91	96	100	105	110	115	119	124	129	134	138	143	148	153	158	162	167
59	94	99	104	109	114	119	124	128	133	138	143	148	153	158	163	168	173
60	97	102	107	112	118	123	128	133	138	143	148	153	158	163	168	174	179
61	100	106	111	116	122	127	132	137	143	148	153	158	164	169	174	180	185
62	104	109	115	120	126	131	136	142	147	153	158	164	169	175	180	186	191
63	107	113	118	124	130	135	141	146	152	158	163	169	175	180	186	191	197
64	110	116	122	128	134	140	145	151	157	163	169	174	180	186	192	197	204
65	114	120	126	132	138	144	150	156	162	168	174	180	186	192	198	204	210
66	118	124	130	136	142	148	155	161	167	173	179	186	192	198	204	210	216
67	121	127	134	140	146	153	159	166	172	178	185	191	198	204	211	217	223
68	125	131	138	144	151	158	164	171	177	184	190	197	203	210	216	223	230
69	128	135	142	149	155	162	169	176	182	189	196	203	209	216	223	230	236
70	132	139	146	153	160	167	174	181	188	195	202	209	216	222	229	236	243
71	136	143	150	157	165	172	179	186	193	200	208	215	222	229	236	243	250
72	140	147	154	162	169	177	184	191	199	206	213	221	228	235	242	250	258
73	144	151	159	166	174	182	189	197	204	212	219	227	235	242	250	257	265
74	148	155	163	171	179	186	194	202	210	218	225	233	241	249	256	264	272
75	152	160	168	176	184	192	200	208	216	224	232	240	248	256	264	272	279
76	156	164	172	180	189	197	205	213	221	230	238	246	254	263	271	279	287

Source: National Institutes of Health, National Heart, Lung, and Blood Institute

not gender specific and has become the measure that most health professionals use because it is more accurate than using weight alone.

BMI is calculated by dividing a person's weight in kilograms (2.2 pounds = 1 kilogram) by height in meters squared. Or, to figure BMI using pounds and inches, multiply your weight in pounds by 700, then divide the result by your height in inches, then divide that result by your height in inches a second time. An easier way is to locate your BMI on the following table.

The NIDDKD has concluded that a BMI of 25 to < 30 is defined as overweight and a BMI of 30 and above as obese. The previous chart indicates waist size as an indicator of risk. Find your waist size on the chart to determine your risk level.

RISK ASSOCIATED DISEASE ACCORDING TO BMI AND WAIST SIZE

BMI		Waist less than or equal to 40 in. (men) or 35 in. (women)	Waist greater than 40 in. (men) or 35 in. (women)
18.5 or less	Underweight	—	N/A
18.5 - 24.9	Normal	—	N/A
25.0 - 29.9	Overweight	Increased	High
30.0 - 34.9	Obese	High	Very High
35.0 - 39.9	Obese	Very High	Very High
40 or greater	Extremely Obese	Extremely High	Extremely High

Source: National Institutes of Health, National Heart, Lung, and Blood Institute

Lifestyle Changes

We know that we are overweight or obese, so what should we do about it? Do we run out and buy the newest fad diet book and follow its instructions? No, we don't think you should diet at all. The word *diet* has shifted from meaning "a way of life" to some "specific way to limit food." Fad diets are just that— fads that we hope go away soon. They do not work, and some of them are dangerous. We want you to approach the food challenge as part of an overall healthy lifestyle. Spend time to learn how to live a healthy lifestyle. It will help you look better, feel better, and may add years to your life.

HEART POINT

Fad diets do not work and some are dangerous.

Calories Count

There is a very simple equation to losing weight: consume fewer calories than your body uses each day. In order to do that, you restrict the total calories consumed and/or you increase the calories used by your body. If we eat more calories than we use up, it is stored as fat (like a bear approaching hibernation). When we store up about 3,500 calories, it accumulates as a pound of fat. Conversely, if you consume fewer calories than the body uses, you start to use up the stored fat. Consume 3,500 fewer calories than the body needs and you lose one pound of fat.

Lose a Pound of Unhealthy Fat per Week

At a steady weight, your body needs the same level of calories every day, or the same average calories, in order to maintain that weight. It takes approximately 15 calories to maintain one pound of body weight. For example, a man who weighs 175 pounds needs about 2,500 calories per day to maintain his weight. As you age you need fewer calories to maintain your weight. Estimate the number of calories you consume each day by maintaining a food log; simply list everything and the amounts of what you consume. This will allow you to determine your daily caloric consumption. In addition, it provides an overview of your eating habits. You can then start to cut certain high-calorie, high-fat foods from your diet, make other choices, or reduce the amount you consume. For instance:

Instead of These Calories	Choose These Calories
1 cup ice cream (270 calories)	8-oz. low-fat, sugar-free yogurt (120 calories)
1 tbsp. butter (100 calories)	spritz nonfat butter flavor spray (0 calories)
8 chocolate chip cookies, 2¼-inch diameter (360 calories)	10 Thompson seedless grapes (35 calories)
3 oz. ground beef patty, broiled (245 calories)	3 oz. tuna, packed, drained (165 calories)
20 potato chips (205 calories)	18 carrot strips (30 calories)
2 tbsp. regular salad dressing (120–170 calories)	2 tbsp. nonfat salad dressing (0 calories)

These are only a small sample of the possible substitutions that can help you move toward healthy living. Each will save you calories and produce other health benefits. You can quickly find savings that add up to 500 calories per day—for example, have a few grapes instead of cookies after dinner and use a nonfat salad dressing instead of regular dressing. If you save 500 calories each day for a week, the total saving is 3,500 calories for that week. That means you will lose one pound. If you continue the same program for one year, you can lose an amazing 52 pounds.

HEART POINT

A British study shows that eating at least six times a day, rather than two large meals, seems to lower cholesterol, even though more fat and total calories were consumed.

It is important for you to understand that taking charge of your life and choosing a healthy lifestyle can produce big rewards. The necessary steps really are not complicated but require consistent effort every day.

Set a Weight-Loss Goal

Many of us want and need to lose a lot of weight, but research suggests that targeting a weight-loss goal of about 10 percent of our body weight in one year is the most achievable goal. It is a level of loss that can be achieved without unusual effort. You are also much more likely to maintain your level once you reach it. Remember that you put the weight on over many years; don't try to take it all off at once.

When to Eat

There is much research on the best times to eat. Perhaps the most-violated rule concerns eating breakfast—more people skip breakfast than any other meal. It may in fact be exactly what Mom told us: "Breakfast is the most important meal of the day." Be sure to allow enough time each morning to enjoy a healthy breakfast. For you "I never have time for breakfast" people, please read in the stress section about planning.

Eat more of your calories in the morning through midday rather than in the evening. The body has more time to use the calories, rather than eating a large meal in the evening, when calories will not be used up prior to going to bed. Those extra calories will be stored as fat.

Many health experts would break meals down from three large meals each day to six or seven smaller meals spread throughout the day. Try to spread your food consumption throughout the day. By consuming a number of small meals throughout the day, you will have fewer and smaller peaks of glucose. That is particularly important for diabetics and those who are glucose impaired.

Create a Food Diary

Keeping a daily diary of all of the food we consume is an automatic reminder to maintain a healthy lifestyle. Add little motivational notes every few pages, or write them on sticky notes, to remind you why you are getting healthy. We have created a form that can be copied and used. There are spaces to record the following: date, time you eat, what you eat, amount eaten, your mood, total fat, saturated fat, cholesterol, and calories. Try to fill in the first part of the list immediately after you eat. You are much more likely to be accurate that way. Use a food encyclopedia as your source and record your fat grams, cholesterol, and calories later. It may be helpful to have a small pocket notepad to record

FOOD DIARY

Date/Time	Food and Amount Consumed	Your Mood	Total Fat	Saturated Fat	Calories	Cholesterol

the same information when you are away from your home. Transfer the information to your food diary when you return home.

Food and Feelings

Eating can be triggered by our emotions. It's important to recognize any eating that you do other than to satisfy hunger. Your food diary has a spot to record how you feel or why you ate. This alerts you to your personal food triggers. Some people overeat because of emotions. They are bored, lonely, depressed, worried, or feel stress from the job or other causes. Some activities trigger people to eat, including when you stop smoking, are tired, eat out, are at a party, work odd hours, or watch TV. Other times you may rationalize or think that you deserve it; it's free; or you are on vacation or at a special occasion. You need to guard against those. Writing down your feelings will make you aware of the reasons you eat.

Portion-Size Chart

You need to be able to estimate accurately how much food you are consuming. The following are some comparisons that will make it easier for you:

Food Serving Size	Equals Size of a Serving	Calories Per Serving	Fat Grams Per Serving
3 oz. meat	deck of cards	225	15
3 oz. fish or poultry	deck of cards	70–110	2
1 oz. cheese	domino	100	8
½ cup pasta	tennis ball	80	1
½ cup grapes	light bulb	60	0
1 cup green salad	baseball	25	0
2 pancakes, plain	(2) 16 oz. cottage-cheese lids	120	0–4
½ cup rice	cupcake wrapper	120	0
4 oz. hamburger patty	lid of a quart mayonnaise jar	320	24
glass of 2% milk	1-cup (8 oz.) measuring cup	120	5

What to Eat

The sections that follow discuss specific categories of food along with our recommendations. There is conflicting information about many of these categories. We help you sort it out to make informed decisions. The suggestions are oriented to anyone with heart disease or anyone at risk.

Fats

Use all fats and oils sparingly. They all are calorie dense, and many are detrimental in other ways. Everyone should understand the main types of fats: saturated, polyunsaturated, and monounsaturated.

Most saturated fats are hard at room temperature or when refrigerated. Animal sources are butter, cheese, cream, whole milk, ice cream, beef, pork, lamb, and poultry skin. Plant sources include coconut oil, palm kernel oil, and palm oil. Consider the hardness of a stick of butter, shortening, or lard; then think of it inside your arteries. In a sense, that is what it does; it clogs your arteries. It also raises your cholesterol level and your risk of heart attack. The average American consumes 14 to 16 percent of their total calories from saturated fats. Never forget the average American diet is killing us. Eliminating saturated fat from your diet would be the healthiest choice possible. The next best thing is to limit consumption to as little as possible.

DARRELL'S STORY

"Before going for my second angiogram, which became my second angioplasty, I was discussing it with my sister. She was curious why I was going back so soon (six weeks). I jokingly replied, 'I think there is a cheeseburger stuck in my artery.' Well, that is pretty close to the truth. Saturated fat from meat, particularly ground beef or hamburgers, along with dairy, whole milk, cheese, etc., is a 'building block' of the plaque that closes down our arteries."

Polyunsaturated fat comes from vegetables and is a better choice than saturated fats. They generally remain in a liquid state at refrigerator temperatures.

Use corn, safflower, soybean, sunflower, cottonseed, and sesame oils sparingly in place of saturated fats. (We listed them in order of preference.)

Monounsaturated fat, and specifically olive oil, is the best choice of all. Though the debate is not fully settled, olive oil seems to provide health benefits to some groups of people. The people in areas near the Mediterranean, who primarily cook with olive oil, have a low incidence of heart attacks and heart disease. Do not forget that olive oil has just as many calories as other oils, about 125 calories per tablespoon, and should be restricted in order to keep weight down. If you are going to consume fats, we recommend sparing use of monounsaturated fat, particularly olive oil.

Hydrogenated fat, partially hydrogenated fat, and all transfats should be avoided. The hydrogenation process hardens liquid oils, which makes them useful for food manufacturing and creating more butter-like margarines. Stick-type margarine contains the most, tub-types less, and semiliquids have the least transfat. They are used in high-fat baked goods, doughnuts, cookies, and cakes. There is even more in French fries and most potato chips, corn chips, and crackers. The transfats are at least as bad as saturated fats in increasing the risk of heart disease and probably much worse. The epidemiologist at the FDA, Kathleen Koehler, Ph.D., suggests a huge benefit for everyone in the United States from removing transfats from margarines and just 3 percent from commercial baked goods. She estimates that it could save 5,000 lives per year, prevent more than 17,000 heart attacks, with a monetary benefit of up to $7.9 billion in savings. Avoid consuming all transfats. Do not eat stick margarine, commercially fried foods, and high-fat baked goods. It is interesting to note that Adelle Davis, perhaps our earliest expert on nutrition and healthy eating, removed all hydrogenated fats from her famous book *Let's Cook It Right* in the 1970 edition, and the FDA is finally catching up.

DARRELL'S STORY

"After I took control of my lifestyle and began eating a very low-fat diet and virtually no meat, I had a conversation with my sister, Linda. In the telephone call she was describing an incident at her daughter, Jennifer's, house. It seems that their cat, Crash, was walking around the kitchen when Jennifer opened the freezer to retrieve something. A frozen package of ground beef slid out and landed on Crash. They rushed Crash to the vet, who treated him for a leg injury. I interrupted my sister and said, 'See, I told you that meat will kill you.' (Crash had a full recovery.)"

Dietary Fat Levels

How much fat should you consume? For most Americans, more than 33 percent of their calories come from fat. There is little or no argument that 33 percent is too much fat. Even this is misleading, because Americans are also eating more food overall and consuming more calories than they used to (which is why we are fatter). The research by Dr. Dean Ornish proves that a vegetarian diet, with 10 percent of calories from fat, combined with exercise and stress reduction can actually reverse blockages in arteries for many patients. Every heart patient and everyone at risk for heart disease needs to know that. Most cardiologists and the AHA do not do enough to educate those at risk so they can make intelligent decisions.

"What we should be doing is removing as much of the saturated fat from our diet as we can. We need to select foods that are lower in total fat and especially in saturated fat," says John E. Vanderveen, Ph.D., director of the Office of Plant and Dairy Foods and Beverages in the FDA's Center for Food Safety and Applied Nutrition.

Is there any safe level of fat consumption above the 10 percent of calories from fat level (Dr. Dean Ornish's recommendation)? The typical Asian diet has only about 10 percent to 20 percent fat, mostly monounsaturated, and they have one of the lowest heart disease rates in the world. The Asian diet includes almost no saturated fat, which is the most dangerous fat to consume. When Asians move to the United States and adopt our typical diet, their heart disease and death rates increase to our levels. When Asians adapt a diet that is between the typical American and Asian diets, their rate of heart disease also increases to levels midway between their old rates and the higher U.S. levels. This research proves a direct link between fat levels consumed and heart disease and death rates. If we cut our fat consumption to the Asian level, 10 percent to 20 percent calories from fat, we will lower our heart disease death rate.

As the amount of fat in our diet increases, so does heart disease. In Dr. Ancel Keys's classic study, detailed in 1958 in the *Annals of Internal Medicine,* comparing the diets and health of Japanese men who migrated from Japan to Hawaii and Los Angeles, the low-fat, traditional diet, with only 10 percent of calories from fat, resulted in low cholesterol levels, averaging 150, and no significant atherosclerosis at any age. With those who migrated to Hawaii and adopted a Polynesian diet, 30 percent of calories came from fat, cholesterol levels rose to 200, and more atherosclerosis resulted. The Japanese

HEART POINT

CALORIC FAT:
Lean Beef—40–60% Fat
Sirloin Steak—85% Fat
Hard Cheese—65–85% Fat
Mayonnaise—100% Fat
Butter—100% Fat

men who moved to Los Angeles and adopted the high-fat diet, with 43 percent of calories from fat, had the worst results of all. Their cholesterol jumped to 240 (the American average at the time of the study), and autopsies showed progressive and severe artery disease.

Diet is a controllable lifestyle choice. You can improve your odds by choosing a low-fat, low-cholesterol diet.

The American Heart Association continues to recommend for the general public total fat of 30 percent of calories in their Step I diet and less in their Step II diets. Many public health agencies recommend similar fat consumption levels. The AHA suggests their revised (in 2000) dietary guidelines help healthy people avoid heart disease. They have recast their information to emphasize eating more fruit, vegetables, and whole grains, along with an added recommendation of two servings of fatty fish (salmon or tuna) per week, and limiting saturated and transfats. It is true that if your current diet has a fat consumption level at 33 percent of calories (current U.S. average) or more, lowering it to 30 percent will improve your odds of avoiding heart disease. With that diet and level of fat, however, more people will be at risk for heart disease than should be. The AHA's recommendations hardly seem adequate based on the heart disease levels of individuals on typical Asian diets and Dr. Ornish's diet. If you can't follow the Ornish program, emulate the Asian diet and keep your total fat consumption between 15 percent to 20 percent calories from fat. It is a much more sensible choice than the AHA's and other public health recommendations. (You should consult a doctor before making any major lifestyle change, including diet. Some individuals with heart disease who are diagnosed with syndrome X—a specific cluster of problems that include high blood pressure, glucose intolerance, excessive abdominal fat, and hyperlipidemia [low HDL cholesterol and high triglycerides]—may not benefit from a low-fat diet.)

Reducing Fat

Most of the fat in our diets comes from, in descending order, meats (including poultry and fish), visible fats (cooking oils and shortening), and dairy products.

HEART POINT

One gram of fat equals 9 calories; it is the most calorie-laden food.

Recent surveys suggest that our fat consumption is about 33 percent of dietary calories from fat. Though this is a lower percentage than in previous years, we have also increased our overall caloric intake. For healthy individuals to remain healthy, they need to cut fat below 30 percent and probably closer to 20 percent calories from fat. Compliance would reduce disease significantly. Heart disease patients and others at risk need to aim for somewhere between 10 percent to 20 percent calories from fat.

To get anywhere near Dr. Ornish's goal of 10 percent calories from fat you need to eliminate all regular dairy products: milk, ice cream, cheese, sour cream, and the rest. There are many no-fat dairy products on the market. Many are terrible, but experiment with different products to find some that are acceptable. Start to make overall changes in your approach. Eat nonfat yogurt rather than ice cream, just a sprinkle of butter-flavored granules or salsa instead of sour cream on your potato, and use nonfat milk on your cereal. Most of the regular, high-fat dairy products are loaded with saturated fat anyway, and you are better off without them. Substitute vegetarian choices for meat-based meals. Use all oils sparingly if at all. There are wonderful nonfat salad dressings on the market. Walden Farms in the eastern United States is one good example. Select one of those instead of regular dressings. Balsamic vinegar also makes a wonderful topping for any salad. Avoid all fried foods and baked goods.

HEART POINT

Fat warning: 2-percent milk (low fat?) has 37 percent of calories from fat.

That leaves us with the meats, the largest amount of fat in our diets. You should eat fatty fish, such as salmon and tuna, from two to four times each week. Fish is much lower in calories than meat, about 25 percent to 50 percent of calories for similar portion, and has added health benefits. The fish and fish oil, including the unsaturated fat Omega-3, helps protect from heart attacks.

Your next best choice is lean, white meat poultry, which is usually lower in fat and calories than other meat. White meat chicken and turkey, cooked without the skin, is the healthiest. A 4-oz. portion of chicken breast without the skin has only 144 calories with 12 percent of the calories from fat.

HEART POINT

FOOD SHOPPING: Never shop when hungry; always have a plan; shop alone; and create a "shopping list form" with low-fat, healthy choices to just fill in.

If you want to have a lifestyle where you consume food that is about 10 percent of the calories from fat, Dr. Ornish's program, you can consume very little fish and poultry each day. A 200-pound man can have about a 2-oz. serving of fish or chicken per day. Remember, though difficult it may be, that diet, combined with exercise and stress reduction, is proven to reverse coronary artery blockages for many people.

As for other meat, you would have to consume even less of it than the chicken and fish to stay within those guidelines. It has far more calories and a higher percentage of calories from fat. So eat meat rarely, if at all, and when you do, select cuts with the least amount of fat.

If you have been a regular meat eater, you will probably have to plan a reduction over time. We know this is not easy, but consider the alternative. Start by trimming all visible fat off meat before cooking. Cut portion size down to a few ounces. We have all heard of restaurants that serve huge portions and huge steaks, 16 oz. to 36 oz. There was even a place that offered to give the customer a second steak if he or she consumed the entire first one, all 36 oz. That is no gift at all. Do they provide transportation to the hospital also?

Calculating Fat as a Percentage of Total Calories

Figuring out your fat calories and percentage of total calories from fat during the day is a bit of work but within the capabilities of anyone with basic math skills and the desire to live a healthy life. Food labels list total fat and saturated fat in grams and as "% Daily Value" for a 2,000-calorie diet. You need to make two conversions to use the nutrition label. The FDA uses 30 percent calories from fat as their guide for "daily value," and that's not really a healthy level.

HEART POINT

Fat warning: "Lean" meat is actually about 40 percent to 50 percent fat; other meats are higher in fat, and ground meat has up to 80 percent of the calories from fat.

Let's start with an example of someone who needs 2,000 calories to maintain a healthy BMI. Twenty percent of the total calories (2,000) is 400 calories from fat per day, divided by 9 calories per gram, totals 44 grams of fat per day. Just add up the fat grams you consume during the course of the day. (Using the Food Diary makes this easier.) If your daily caloric intake to maintain a healthy BMI is 1,500 calories, your total fat grams for the day equals 33 (1,500 x 0.20, divided by 9).

A quarter-pound cheeseburger at a typical fast food restaurant may have from 32 fat grams to 42 fat grams, a regular-size French fries 12 fat grams, a plain baked potato 2 fat grams, but add sour cream and the total is 15 grams of fat.

Fruits and Vegetables

There is virtually total agreement that if we all consumed more—a lot more in some cases—fruits and vegetables we would be much healthier. Hundreds of studies support the consumption of fruit and vegetables. Individuals who eat from three to five servings per day show a lower risk of high blood pressure, less risk of coronary heart disease, and a lower risk of ischemic stroke than those who consume fewer servings. Some studies support eating as many as ten servings per day. In addition, there is lots of evidence that eating fruit and vegetables lowers the risk of many forms of cancer.

Most fruits and vegetables are naturally very low in fat and cholesterol. (Beware of the exceptions: coconuts, avocados, and olives, which are high in fat. Consider them as fats.) Many are high in fiber. Perhaps best of all, many have wonderful flavor, are naturally sweet, and have great "mouth feel," so are very satisfying and filling. The food guide pyramid lists the following recommended servings: fruit, two to four; vegetables, three to five. Heart patients should always eat four servings of fruit and five or more servings of vegetables each day.

Fiber

Fiber comes from the cell walls of plants and provides the bulk to move waste out of our bodies. High-fiber foods are generally foods consumed in a natural, unprocessed state. There are two different forms of fiber named and defined by their solubility in water.

Soluble fiber absorbs water, acting like a sponge. That swelling creates bulk in your stomach and slows food absorption. It helps you feel more satisfied with the food you eat. It also forms a gel with cholesterol and triglycerides

HEART POINT

Fill most of your plate with vegetables before any other category of food.

HEART POINT

FRUIT AND VEGETABLE SERVING SIZE: One serving equals a medium-size piece of fruit, a cup of raw leafy vegetables, ½ cup cooked vegetables, or 6 oz. of juice.

and carries some of them out of your body rather than being absorbed into the bloodstream. Good sources of soluble fiber include grapefruit, oranges, strawberries, whole oats, oat bran, beans, and peas.

Insoluble fiber, such as wheat bran, does not dissolve in water and helps move waste through our intestines. Researchers suggest that this quick movement of waste through our bodies reduces the risk of colon cancer and may help related problems like diverticulosis and hemorrhoids. Good sources of insoluble fiber include Brussels sprouts, cabbage, carrots, cauliflower, whole wheat bread, and wheat bran. Most foods that have fiber have both soluble and insoluble fiber. People eating high-fiber diets seem to take longer to eat and feel more sated, both useful in maintaining a healthy lifestyle and weight.

HEART POINT

Equivalent serving sizes: Bread—1 slice or 1 oz.; ½ hamburger bun; 4 to 6 crackers; ½ cup cooked cereal, potato, or pasta; ⅓ cup rice; ¾ cup cereal; ½ cup cooked beans; ½ cup sweet potato, yam, corn, or peas.

The average American consumes about 10 grams of fiber per day. The National Cancer Institute recommends eating a minimum of five servings of fruit and vegetables each day, a good start toward their recommended 20 to 35 grams of fiber. Even better would be to increase fruit and vegetable consumption and add whole grains, about six servings per day, and beans to your diet.

A recent study published in the *Archives of Internal Medicine* encourages the consumption of beans. The results showed that when individuals consumed legumes four or more times per week they reduced their risk of coronary artery disease by 22 percent compared with those who consumed legumes less than once a week. The study looked at various dry beans, pinto beans, red beans, black-eyed peas, plus peanuts and peanut butter.

High-fat foods, sugar, and highly refined foods elevate insulin in the body, which contributes to weight gain. High-fiber, low-fat foods and lowering total caloric consumption do the opposite—they decrease insulin in the body and slow absorption of glucose into the system. It is particularly important for diabetics to combine consumption of high-fiber and low-fat foods, along with regular exercise.

Water

Water is so basic it feels strange to be reminded of its importance to health and a healthy lifestyle. We were always taught that eight 8-oz. glasses of water were needed each day. It is critical for a healthy lifestyle to consume at least that amount of water. Drink water throughout the day. Have one full glass of water about thirty minutes before meals. That will help "fill you up" so you will not be so hungry. As you exercise more, increase water consumption in proportion, being careful to avoid dehydration. Drink water before, during, and after exercise. For every 8 oz. of coffee or other caffeinated beverage consumed, drink an additional equal amount of water. Caffeine is a diuretic, which rids the body of water. It's not important whether the water comes from the tap or a bottle, sparkling or not, as long as the water is safe for human consumption. Flavored water is also fine as long as it isn't sweetened, which will add needless calories. Add a slice of lemon or lime to water for quick flavor. Bottled water is a convenient way to have water with you any place or time you need it. During exercise and summer increase consumption to replace moisture lost through sweating. Do not consume sodas or other flavored, sugared beverages in place of water. Some also contain caffeine along with sugar and hundreds of calories.

DARRELL'S STORY

"A relative of mine, name left out to protect the guilty, is one of the few people I know who lost weight in her first five months of pregnancy. Her doctor told her to stop drinking soda pop because the caffeine is not good for the baby. She gave up her eight to ten cans per day, saving almost 1,000 calories every single day, losing almost twenty pounds during those five months, and then started to add typical pregnancy pounds. I'm happy to report that mom and new baby are doing fine, except she is back drinking soda and adding the pounds back on."

Cut Sodium (Salt) Use

Over the years there has been much discussion about salt use and its effect on high blood pressure. The average American consumes about 3,600 milligrams of sodium per day compared with a general health recommendation to limit consumption to 2,400 milligrams per day.

A recent study of over 450 individuals showed that you can reduce blood pressure by following a healthy diet, the DASH (Dietary Approach to Stop Hypertension) diet. The DASH diet is lower in fat, saturated fat, cholesterol, and sweets, but with plenty of fruits and vegetables. The individuals on the DASH diet reduced their blood pressure, but those who also controlled their sodium intake to less than 1,500 milligrams had the largest drop in blood pressure. Many heart patients also battle high blood pressure and would benefit from a lifestyle reduction in salt.

To cut salt use:

♦ Don't add salt when cooking. Put your saltshakers away.
♦ Add herbs and spice in place of salt; fresh herbs are better than dry.
♦ If you use canned vegetables or beans, rinse them in water before use.
♦ Avoid eating processed foods and snacks, which are high in salt.
♦ Concentrate on eating fresh fruits and vegetables.

Cut Sugar Use

Sugar is high in calories and immediately affects the body, giving us that "sugar high or buzz." This quickly throws our body's glucose levels into higher numbers. That's harmful for everyone but particularly so for diabetics.

Americans are now eating between 20 to 34 "added" teaspoons of sugar every day. The term *added* refers to sugar that is over and above what is naturally contained in food such as fruit. The food pyramid and guidelines suggest that someone on a 2,200 calorie-per-day diet should consume "only" 12 teaspoons of sugar.

Individuals who consume higher levels of sugar also consume higher total calories, yet have a poor intake of other nutrients, including vitamins A, E, C, all the B vitamins, magnesium, iron, zinc, and calcium. Even worse, the difference in those who consume the highest and lowest amounts of added sugar is about 190 calories a day—which translates into a weight gain of twenty pounds per year. In order to stay healthy and avoid obesity, consume as few added sugars as possible.

Watch out for "hidden" sugars in processed food (again, eat as little as possible). The labels refer to them by their many names. Table sugar is sucrose; other sugars include glucose (dextrose), fructose (levulose), and lactose. There are also the sugar alcohols: sorbitol, xylitol, and mannitol, which, along with fructose, have less effect on blood glucose levels than table sugar. Beet sugar, brown sugar, cane sugar, confectioner's sugar, maple syrup, raw sugar, and turbinado are sucrose in different forms. Carob powder, corn syrup, starch syrup, sugar cane syrup, sweetened condensed milk, and chocolate are all very high in sugar, some also in fat.

HEART POINT

SUGAR HIGH: Sugar consumption is now 30 percent higher than in 1983. USDA figures estimate we use 158 pounds of sugar per year per person in the United States.

Artificial Sweeteners

The American Diabetes Association says that diabetics can use artificial sweeteners in moderate amounts. Saccharin is 300 times sweeter than sugar and can be used in cold and hot foods. Be aware that a very large amount of saccharin causes cancer in laboratory animals. Human studies suggest that it does not cause cancer in people. Aspartame (NutraSweet®) is 180 times sweeter than sugar. It does have calories, but because you need only a tiny amount, it adds few calories to your recipes. You can't use it in baked goods because it loses its sweetness when heated. It can be added to things like pudding at the end of cooking. Acesulfame potassium (Sweet One®), or acesulfame-K is new to the market and can be used in cooking and baking. It doesn't break down when heated, but the texture of baked goods is different than with sugar. Sucralose (Splenda®), 600 times as sweet as sugar, is the newest of the sugar replacements. It cannot be metabolized by your body so passes through your system. It can be used in baking.

Vitamins and Supplements

There continues to be much debate about vitamins and supplements. There is little actual proof from medical studies that shows that we should or should not take them. There is research that hints at negative effects from large doses of antioxidants, but much more needs to be done before proof is available. There is also little chance of harm with reasonable dosage levels, but because of possible interactions you should always review all vitamin and supplement usage with each of your doctors. Discuss any new vitamin or supplement with them before you start taking it. Only 40 percent of the 24 million people taking supplements discuss the fact with their doctors. Most doctors have little background in herbal supplements. Both of you can stay informed through a new online database from the National Institutes of Health devoted to supplements (www//odp.od.nih.gov/ods/databases/ibids.html) that provides an up-to-date bibliography of the latest research.

There are two distinct camps in the vitamin disagreement. One group suggests that if you eat a decent diet, you will get all of the vitamins you need. Dr. Kenneth Cooper unofficially leads the group that suggests that you need a range of the antioxidant vitamins to protect your arteries from the damage of free radicals (volatile molecules that some experts suggest cause chemical damage and injure cells and DNA). He goes on to suggest that an antioxidant regimen will reduce the risk of heart disease, cancer, cataracts, and delay premature aging. He recommends larger daily dosages than the FDA minimum daily requirements and for those who are heavier, men, and those who exercise vigorously. He suggests the following: vitamin C—500–3,000 mg; Vitamin E (natural forms)—200–1,200 IU; beta-carotene—10,000–50,000 IU; selenium—50–100 mcg. Those on blood thinners (aspirin, Coumadin, and others) should be very careful with vitamin E, which also thins the blood. It also may raise blood pressure.

DARRELL'S STORY

"In addition to the antioxidants, I also take the following supplements: B-complex (vitamin B6—100 mg, vitamin B12—100 mcg, folic acid—

400 mcg) to help regulate homocysteine levels; GTF chromium—200 mcg, and fenugreek—610 mg twice a day to help blood glucose levels; and coenzyme Q10—120 mg to replace coenzyme Q10 my body cannot make because of prescription drugs. Coenzyme Q10 may also help before heart surgery in addition to angina, heart failure, and gum disease."

Healthy Cooking Methods

Learn to use the healthiest cooking methods and equipment. Use high-quality nonstick cookware to avoid using fats. Try a Crock-Pot for slow-cooking soups. Stir-fry (the only frying you should ever do) in a seasoned Chinese wok with a tiny bit of peanut oil. Other preparation techniques include:

♦ Bake using tightly covered cookware. Add extra liquid if necessary.
♦ Stew or braise in similar cookware with more liquid, either on stovetop or in oven. Remove fat after refrigerating and before reheating.
♦ Poach in wine, water, or low-fat liquid (good for chicken and fish).
♦ Grill, indoors or out, or broil (good for chicken, fish, and vegetables).

QUICK AND EASY FRUIT AND VEGETABLES

♦ Eat salad for lunch or dinner; add a variety of chopped vegetables; use nonfat dressing.
♦ Have vegetable snacks on hand all the time. Try baby carrots, bell pepper rings, broccoli florets, cauliflower florets, cherry tomatoes, and celery sticks; keep them in zipper bags in the refrigerator.
♦ Use fresh fruit for snacks. Apples, bananas, grapes, and pears are tasty and portable. Try frozen grapes in the summer.
♦ Add chopped vegetables to broth-type soups and pasta. Broccoli, carrots, yellow, red, and green peppers, mushrooms and zucchini add flavor and color.

- Microwave almost anything, requires no extra fat; fast also.
- Steam vegetables in a basket (steamer) over boiling water.

Recipes

Darrell has been working on his favorite recipes to rid them of fat and calories. (We have listed some good cookbooks with healthy recipes in the bibliography.) The two that follow have plenty of flavor and nutrition without much fat:

SUBSTITUTIONS TO SAVE CALORIES AND FAT

RECIPE CALLS FOR:	LOW (NO)-FAT SUBSTITUTE:
Buttermilk	Nonfat or low-fat buttermilk, or nonfat yogurt
Butter	Oil, fruit purees or combination, silken tofu, potato or sweet potato puree
Chocolate	Cocoa powder; 2 tbsp. for each oz.
Cheese	Nonfat or low-fat cheese
Cream cheese	Fat-free cream cheese
Egg	2 egg whites for 1 egg, or egg substitute
Heavy cream	Evaporated skim milk or half amount each low-fat yogurt and low-fat cottage cheese
Oil	Fruit puree or use less oil with fruit puree; silken tofu, potato, or sweet potato puree; applesauce or bananas
Salt	Reduce by two-thirds or eliminate; add herbs and spices
Sour cream	Fat-free plain yogurt; low-fat cottage cheese (blended); nonfat or low-fat sour cream
Whole milk	Skim milk or nonfat milk

DARRELL'S WHOLE WHEAT PANCAKES
Makes about eight 4-inch pancakes

¾ cup stone-ground whole wheat flour
1 tsp. baking powder
2 tsp. sugar
1 egg yolk
3 egg whites
¾ (scant) nonfat milk

Mix the dry ingredients together in a bowl large enough for the complete recipe. Separate 3 eggs; put whites into a large copper or stainless-steel mixing bowl; add 1 yoke to the dry ingredients. Add milk to dry ingredients, mix quickly with a fork, about 20 strokes. Don't overmix. Start to prewarm griddle. Whisk the egg whites to soft peaks (kids like this noisy method) or use an electric mixer. Using a large rubber spatula, scrape the whites into the mixed ingredients and then fold in. Spray griddle with nonstick butter-flavored spray. When water drops skip across griddle it is ready for use. Ladle ¼ cup* of batter onto griddle. When bubbles appear and then pop open, turn the pancakes over. When the other side is cooked, serve immediately on warmed plate.

Top with I Can't Believe It's Not Butter® spray (no fat, yet good flavor) and preserves, fresh fruit, or syrup.

*I use a ¼-cup size measuring cup with a handle for measuring flour, then batter.

DARRELL'S STORY

"I made pancakes almost every Saturday for thirty years. They were wonderful (if I don't say so myself), though they were actually quite high in fat and low in nutrition. The basic recipe came from *Joy of Cooking*, my basic cooking guide. I managed to add some fat, particularly on the griddle, then more butter on top of them, and lots of syrup. They were made with highly processed white flour. After bypass surgery I knew I had to reform and improve my lifestyle, including eating and cooking. To improve my pancakes I switched to whole wheat flour, left out the fat, the eggs, and the sugar—result; they were simply awful. Then I started to rework my approach and created the preceding recipe, which is healthy and tasty."

VEGETARIAN PARTY CHILI
Makes 20 1-cup servings

3 large peppers (green, red, or yellow; mixed is ideal), chopped

1 lb. carrots, scrubbed and chopped

3 cups chopped onion

2 tbsp. olive oil

4 cloves garlic, minced

1 16-oz. bag dry black beans (about 5 cups cooked beans), or use 2 16-oz. cans black beans

1 16-oz. can dark red kidney beans (rinsed)

1 16-oz. can cranberry beans (rinsed)

1 28-oz. can crushed tomatoes (ones with good texture, less salt)

1 6-oz. can tomato paste

3 tbsp. chili powder

1 tbsp. oregano

1 bunch fresh cilantro, chopped

2 tbsp. cumin

Chop peppers (about 1-inch x 1-inch pieces), carrots (about ½-inch x ¼-inch pieces), and onion (about ½-inch x ¼-inch pieces). Coat vegetables with oil, then add ½ cup of water and cook until somewhat tender. Turn off heat, add minced garlic. Rinse canned beans, add to cooked beans. Add vegetables, crushed tomatoes, tomato paste, chili powder, and oregano to the beans. Mix and simmer for 30 minutes. Add a little water as needed. Immediately before serving add chopped cilantro and cumin.

NOTE: *Part of the success of this chili is the final color and texture, so you want a variety of peppers and beans with texture. Do not overcook them.*

Preparing dry beans

Rinse dry beans, sort, then cover with four times the water and bring to a boil. Reduce to simmer for three minutes, then let stand, tightly covered, for one hour. Change water, then bring to simmer and cook until tender, drain. (Allow 2½ to 3 hours for this.)

Cleaning cilantro

Fresh cilantro is fabulous but almost always full of sand. Clean by submerging and soaking cilantro in a large quantity of cool water. Shake it occasionally and change water three to four times. You will know it is clean when you find no more sand on the bottom of the soaking container.

Spiciness

To my taste, this is not a "spicy" chili. Adjust the recipe to your own personal taste, adding as much chili powder and cumin as you desire.

QUIT SMOKING, THE KILLER HABIT

SMOKING IS A terrible habit. Even most of those who smoke would agree that it's not something someone should start and it would be better if they stopped. It is one of the top two causes of preventable death in the United States. (Obesity has been moving up fast and will soon exceed it.) Smoking causes more than 500,000 deaths from cancer, heart disease, respiratory disease, plus injuries and death from smoking-related fires. Think of the public uproar and call for action if four 747s crashed every day for a year, 1,315 fatal crashes. The total death toll would equal the preventable deaths caused by smoking.

Smoking is a "dose-specific" killer. The more years you smoke, the more cigarettes per day you smoke, and the amount of nicotine, tar, and carbon monoxide contained in each cigarette determine your risk of heart disease. Depending on what age you start to smoke, each cigarette you smoke will cut your life by fifteen to twenty seconds.

EATING TO LIVE POINTS

- ◆ Enjoy cooking and eating.
- ◆ Cut 500 calories per day out of your diet until you reach a healthy level.
- ◆ Consume as little fat as possible, 20 percent of calories or less.
- ◆ Use monounsaturated fat sparingly when you use fat.
- ◆ Consume no transfats.
- ◆ Search for low-fat foods you love.
- ◆ Eat lots of fruit and vegetables, nine servings per day or more.
- ◆ Consume mostly whole, not processed, grains.
- ◆ Exercise at least thirty minutes daily.
- ◆ Eat only when hungry and for no other reason.
- ◆ Consume as little added sugar as possible.
- ◆ Cut sodium consumption.
- ◆ Get weight down to a healthy level, a BMI under 25.
- ◆ Aim to lose no more than 10 percent of your body weight each year.
- ◆ Build a healthy lifestyle support structure of family, friends, and colleagues.
- ◆ Drink at least eight 8-oz. glasses of pure water daily.
- ◆ Take charge of your lifestyle and eat to live.

Smoking and Heart Disease

There are 4,000 chemicals and compounds in cigarette smoke, and many are toxic. Some of the gases in smoke include ammonia, nitric acid, acetone, carbon monoxide, and cyanide. Most of those gases would be labeled with a skull and crossbones if they were held in a container. The tar you inhale creates more than a dozen carcinogens, including ammonia and nicotine. Nicotine cranks heart rate up fifteen to twenty-five beats per minute and blood pressure ten to twenty points. Carbon monoxide displaces oxygen and injures artery walls. Just as the heart and blood pressure kick up higher, there is less oxygen available, which strains the heart muscle. That can produce a heart attack.

HEART POINT

A two-pack-a-day smoker loses 8.3 years of his life by smoking, more years if he also has coronary artery disease.

DARRELL'S STORY

"As I write this book, my father suffers with emphysema. His health has deteriorated over the last few years until he uses a number of inhalers, medicine delivered through a nebulizer, a breathing device, and needs to be on oxygen twenty-four hours per day. He is no longer able to drive, is weak and able to walk very short distances only, and eating tires him out. There is nothing we can do—it is very difficult to watch. He smoked two to three packs of cigarettes each day of his life from the time he was a teenager. He is so hooked on this terrible drug that he still cannot give it up and smokes about a half a pack per day, even as it has left him with less than 19 percent of his lung capacity."

HEART POINT

A pack-a-day smoking habit sends one cup of tar into your lungs each year.

Passive Smoke

Nonsmokers are also at risk. Anyone in a home with a smoker will also have damage from passive smoke. Infants and children exposed to smoke in the home have a higher chance of ear infections, asthma, respiratory damage, and persistent coughs. Studies show that lung development is impaired, and there may be an impact on mental and behavioral development. Insist that smokers smoke someplace else, not inside your home or air space.

Prepare to Quit

You have to weigh all the facts and must choose to quit; you must commit. We know it's not easy and will not lie to you, but you can do it. More than 3 million Americans stop smoking every year. Figure out why you want to do it and make a list of all of the reasons. Repeat one of those reasons to yourself each morning and night. In addition to the logical health reasons to quit, think of personal reasons to stop. For example, think of your "smoker-breath," clothes and car odor, all the time wasted taking smoke breaks, and think of your children or grandchildren. Prepare to quit by getting plenty of rest; drinking more fluids; and starting a moderate exercise program. Pick a specific day to quit. It might be easier to pick some special day in your life, such as your anniversary, birthday, or the Great American Smokeout. You will have even more to celebrate in future years, and it will be easy to track your success. Think and read about various ways to quit and select what will work best for you.

HEART POINT

The average age a two-pack-a-day smoker suffers his or her first heart attack—51.

Gradually Cut Back

Find ways to smoke less. Try smoking only half of each cigarette or smoking only during half of the hours of the day, say only the odd or even hours. Set a quota of how many you will smoke each day, and for each cigarette over that amount donate $1.00 to the American Cancer Society or a local charity. Switch to a brand that you dislike or one that is low in tar and nicotine, though don't smoke more of them or more deeply. Cut down to seven cigarettes a day, then set a quit date.

When You Quit

The day that you quit plan lots of activities, such as going to the movies, gardening, taking walks, or riding a bike. Plan to stay busy for several weeks. Plan to have your teeth cleaned to get rid of the tobacco stains—think how nice they are and how much you want to keep them that way. Think of a way to treat yourself for your success and for saving on the cost of cigarettes. Let your family and friends know you are quitting and ask for their help. Even better, get someone else to quit at the same time.

Throw away all cigarettes, matches, lighters, and ashtrays. Wash your clothes and get as much smoke out of them as possible. Clean up your environment, now smoke-free, at home and work. Bring in scented, fresh flowers. They not only will smell better than they have in years, but also will improve your attitude. Hang "no smoking" signs on the doors to your house or apartment and in your car. Don't let others smoke in those places. Warn anyone who is about to visit your house that it is a now a no-smoking zone.

Plan to spend as much time as possible in smoke-free places such as museums, libraries, and theaters. Avoid coffee, alcohol, or other drinks you associate with cigarettes and drink lots of water, juice, or other noncaffeinated beverages. If you miss the sensation of something in your hand or mouth, use replacements. Try pencils or paper clips in your hand. For your mouth use a toothpick, carrots, celery, apples, or sugarless gum.

Withdrawal Symptoms

Smoking is an addiction that some suggest is as bad as heroin or cocaine. There are going to be physical withdrawal symptoms; your body still craves nicotine. Get as much support as possible and use every trick at your disposal. For some patients, that may not be enough. Consult your doctor about prescriptions available. There are nicotine patches, chewing gum, and antidepressants. They may be right for you.

DARRELL'S STORY

"I stopped smoking my pipe over twelve years ago. I had chain-smoked, pipe after pipe, for over twenty-five years. I had foolishly started in college to look 'cool.' I really had no intention of quitting until my wife, Geri, came home from her doctor diagnosed with asthma and an order from her doctor for me to quit. I knew I had no choice and planned my approach. I smoked the last of my pipe tobacco and quit 'cold turkey.' I used no drugs or support groups. I was miserable and difficult to live with for over eight weeks, but I succeeded. I have never smoked since that day, and I'm grateful."

The withdrawal symptoms are strongest the first few weeks. Some people suggest that the symptoms may last only a couple of weeks, but most people have a longer withdrawal. They will diminish after that, but some urge for a cigarette may be with you for years. Be prepared to fight that urge. A stressful event in the future may also trigger your desire to smoke; resist that also. It may even be a good idea to enlist a good friend, who is also a reformed smoker, in a "mutual aid society." Call each other whenever you have a significant urge to smoke and talk each other out of it.

ALEX'S STORY
(heart patient, 55)

"I smoked a minimum of three packs of cigarettes a day for about thirty years. Along with stress, it was my major risk factor for heart disease. In the hospital, after the heart attack, I realized I had to stop smoking. I can't do anything in moderation, so I got some help from drugs. Withdrawal is extraordinarily difficult, with depression-like symptoms.

The drugs help you through that. I felt awful. It's about time doctors understood how difficult it is and show patients some sensitivity."

Avoiding Weight Gain

Most people use "gaining weight" as the reason they won't stop smoking. You can stop smoking and not gain weight, or at least minimize the weight gain. Removing nicotine does lower your basal metabolism rate (BMR) as much as 200 calories per day. Some people also increase their food consumption because of the added stress of withdrawal.

Plan to get more exercise each day. That will help raise your BMR, improve your mood, and simply keep you busy and your mind off quitting. Plan on lots of crunchy foods, like celery, apples, and carrots, to keep your mouth busy and your tummy full. Drink at least eight full glasses of water each day. It's also a good idea to work on improving your diet before quitting cigarettes.

What If I Relapse?

It is possible that you will not succeed quitting the first time, or even a second or third time. Just do not give up trying. Again, the only failure is not trying. The health benefits of not smoking are so great you must keep at it.

EXERCISE

"The wise, for cure, on exercise depend."
—JOHN DRYDEN, *Epistles* (1700)

WE HAVE ALREADY looked at stress reduction and healthy eating as parts of a personal plan to *Surviving with Heart.* Most authorities agree that a diet low in fat, cholesterol, and sodium, in combination with aerobic exercise and stress reduction, will produce substantial benefits for all heart and cardiovascular disease patients, plus many others.

Exercise is a major component of a healthy lifestyle. If you currently lead a sedentary life, you need to learn to move and incorporate regular vigorous activities into your life. If you already do some exercise you may want to do more and get more benefits. Exercise is a "dose-specific" prescription—the more you do the more benefits you gain. Exercise helps control your weight and gives you a sense of accomplishment. It improves how you feel mentally and physically. If there were a single pill that did that, the medical establishment would hail it as the greatest medical breakthrough of all time.

What Exercise Does for You

You already know that exercise helps to reduce stress and improve mental attitude. However, what does it do for the body, and how much exercise do you need to do every day in order to benefit? Research published in the *New England Journal of Medicine* concludes that as little as one-and-a-half hours of vigorous exercise (jogging, aerobics, etc.) per week will significantly help individuals to avoid heart disease. Even just briskly walking (a twenty-minute-per-mile pace or faster) for three hours per week will provide similar results. Even walking as little as one hour a week produces a 30 percent reduction in heart attacks and deaths from other coronary problems.

You can tell from the opening remarks in this section that even a small amount of exercise is good for you and certainly better than a sedentary lifestyle. A balanced program, including exercise of longer duration, would be better yet. The same is true for exercise intensity. For instance, walking faster or jogging, instead of walking over the same time spans, produces greater benefits for the heart (though jogging and other high-impact activities may not be best for everyone).

Later in this Star Point we give specific examples of what types of exercise you might do and how each benefits you. Perhaps the most important thing is to find some activity that you enjoy. If you do it because you love it, it will seem easy and you are much more likely to make it a lifelong habit. If you enjoy gardening, swimming, and biking, just do them on a regular basis. We also encourage everyone to walk. It is an easy, safe, low-cost activity that virtually everyone can do and enjoy. We encourage you to do all of these activities with friends, relatives, and caregivers. Exercising together gives you time to socialize and release stress by having fun together.

Feeling and Looking Better

We discuss the long-term benefits of exercise, particularly the cardiovascular improvements that lower your risk profile for heart attack, strokes, and other complications, later in this Star Point. While the long-term benefits are measurable with specific physical tests and criteria, the quickest reward is how you feel. As you integrate a regular exercise program into your life, you will start to feel and look better. That is a major personal reward. Sagging muscles will start to firm, and your belly, butt, or other problem spots will get smaller and firmer. Your clothes will fit again. You will have more energy for other fun activities such as playing with grandchildren, hiking, or sex. As you start to look and feel better, you will have more self-confidence. Your more attractive body will give you a better self-image. Yes, your cardiologist will measure your improvements in minutes on the treadmill, but you will already know you are healthier. Can you think of a better personal reward than feeling and looking better? We don't think so.

Heart Benefits of Exercise

> *"Health is the vital principle of bliss,*
> *And exercise, of health."*
>
> —JAMES THOMSON, *The Castle of Indolence* (CANTO I, STANZA 55)

Those patients with cardiovascular disease will be most interested in what exercise does for the cardiovascular system and how it affects the underlying risk factors of heart disease. The heart is a muscle and, like other muscles throughout your body, gets stronger with exercise. As the heart gets stronger, it has to work less to pump the oxygenated blood throughout your body. A stronger heart has a lower resting heart rate. A well-conditioned heart will be under less strain when called on to supply blood during any strenuous activity.

Many doctors believe that exercise promotes the growth of new blood vessels, collateral arteries, to the heart. As yet, there is no conclusive proof that collateral circulation develops because of exercise, but it is a wonderful possibility. This is sort of a "natural bypass" for those with blockages, enough to lower the risk of a heart attack. Exercise also helps to lower triglycerides and LDL cholesterol, the "lousy cholesterol," and raise HDL cholesterol, the "healthy cholesterol."

DARRELL'S STORY

"When I had my first angioplasty, my left anterior descending artery was 100 percent closed. The blockage was substantial and in place for some time. I had undiagnosed angina for over five months. My surgeon told me that my collateral arteries kept the blood flowing and helped prevent a heart attack. I had been walking four miles a day, four to five days per week, at aerobic pace. I believe exercise helped me avoid a heart attack."

Exercise improves blood sugar control for Type II diabetics. That could mean fewer prescription medications or lower dosages and fewer complications from uncontrolled blood sugar. A recent study at Duke University Medical Center showed that intensive, long-term exercise helps the body control blood sugar levels. That benefit continued for a full month after exercise was stopped. It also lowers your LDL cholesterol and blood pressure, which lessens the damage inside your arteries. Those benefits all reduce the risk of coronary artery disease, angina, heart attack, and stroke.

Exercise also improves your lung capacity and strengthens your bones, ligaments, and tendons, particularly important as we age and for women after menopause. Exercise also lowers your risk of osteoporosis.

Regression of Heart Disease with Exercise

Research has confirmed that exercise can actually produce regression of coronary artery disease (CAD) for some individuals. Dr. R. Hambrecht, and colleagues, reporting in the *Journal of the American College of Cardiology* (vol. 22, 1993), showed the effect of physical activity on CAD lesions in a controlled and randomized trial. More than 25 percent of the patients in the study, with an expenditure of 2,200 calories per week, achieved a reversal. An expenditure of 1,530 calories stopped the progression of disease.

DARRELL'S STORY

"I try to walk a bit faster than four miles per hour for sixty minutes each outing in a hilly park five days per week. I estimate that activity uses about 2,450 calories per week. That level of exercise combined with a low-fat diet improves my odds considerably."

Exercise and Your Mind

We have known for years the physical benefits of exercise but recently have also learned that exercise benefits our minds. The Institute for the Study of Aging and the International Longevity Center–USA recommends exercise as one way to keep our minds working as well as possible as we age, maybe even into our nineties and older. You should also cut back on caffeine and alcohol and totally avoid tobacco smoke, all of which have a negative impact on blood flow to the brain or kill brain cells and are bad for the heart and coronary arteries.

Clinical depression is a significant problem for many patients after bypass surgery or after a heart attack. Exercise reduces depression for healthy older men, cardiac patients, and those with depression. Individuals who are active, rather than sedentary, are much less likely to have symptoms of anxiety and depression. Those who begin to exercise also show a significant improvement in overall psychological functioning.

Exercise and Burning Calories

In the last section, we looked at healthy eating and reducing calorie intake to bring our weight and BMI down to healthy levels. We showed how cutting 500 calories per day from your food consumption (3,500 calories per week) will help you lose about a pound per week, or as much as 52 pounds in a year.

Let's look at what increasing our activity levels will do for our weight. We use walking as an example. If you walked for thirty minutes at a slow, 2-to-2.5-miles-per-hour pace, you would use 104 calories if you weigh 130 pounds or 160 calories if you weigh 200 pounds. If you walk four times per week, the total calories used would be 416 and 624 respectively. If you picked the pace up a bit and walked at 3.5 miles per hour, you would use 156 and 240 calories per day and 624 and 960 per week. At that pace, you would lose a little over

9 pounds and 14 pounds per year respectively. This just points out that even a small amount of exercise helps you to lose weight or to keep it off.

CALORIES BURNED

EXERCISE	PACE	WEIGHT (130 LBS.) (4x/WK)	WEIGHT (200 LBS.) (4x/WK)
Walk 30 min.	2.5 mph	104 calories (416)	160 calories (640)
Walk 30 min.	3.5 mph	156 calories (624)	240 calories (960)

Basal Metabolic Rate (BMR)

In truth, it is a bit more complicated than just cutting calories. Our bodies need a certain number of calories to take care of our basic needs such as maintaining our body temperature (this takes place at our cellular level). This is called our basal metabolic rate (BMR) and uses about 1,400 calories per day for an average-size person. People have different BMRs because they have different amounts of lean body tissue. The more lean body tissue you have the higher your BMR. Conversely, if you have more fat, you will have a lower BMR. Men tend to have a higher BMR than women because they have more lean muscle tissue. We all lose muscle tissue as we age. Between the age of forty-five and sixty-five, people can lose 15 percent of their muscle mass. This loss lowers their BMR. If they do not increase their exercise levels and continue to eat the same way they always have, their BMR will decrease and they will gain weight. That is what happens to most individuals.

When people reduce their caloric intake to lose weight, their BMR also decreases. This is our body's way of trying to survive. Think of a starving person, which is really what you are when you cut your caloric intake to lose weight. The body reacts and slows down all possible internal organs to save energy. The only way to overcome this change is to exercise. Exercise actually increases your BMR, rather than allowing it to decrease. The higher BMR also continues for four to seven hours after you have finished exercising. Therefore it's just not the calories we burn during exercise, but the increase in our BMR, that provides benefits over a longer time period. That is why it is necessary to exercise if you want to lose weight. Studies show that the most successful weight-loss efforts include exercise. As you lose fat and add lean muscle tissue, your BMR also increases. If you are in better shape and maintain that lean muscle tissue, your BMR will stay permanently at the higher level.

How Much Exercise Is Enough?

You have noticed in this Star Point that various levels and intensities of exercise are useful for various individuals. Usually, the greater duration and intensity of the exercise, the better it is for your health. The best recommendations for exercise levels for heart health are provided by epidemiologist Dr. Ralph S. Paffenbarger, Jr., who has extensively studied the relationship between exercise and heart disease. Based on his research, he suggested that heart attack rates decline progressively starting at activity levels that burn 500 to 999 calories per week. The incidence of heart attacks continues to decline until the 2,000-calorie-per-week level. A 150-pound person walking for forty-five minutes per day at four miles per hour for five days per week uses 1,305 calories. If that person walked at the same pace for sixty minutes each of the five days he or she would use 1,740 calories.

HEART POINT

Turn your daily walk into a goal. Darrell says, "This year I am going to walk from New York City to Nashville. If I walk 25 miles per week and the total distance is 902 miles, it will take about thirty-six weeks to make my goal."

Diabetics and Exercise

Diabetics should monitor and control blood glucose all of the time. Exercise creates extra demands on the body and affects blood sugar readings. Exercise can act much like oral medications that lower blood sugar. You need to plan exercise around meals, snacks, and medication times. As you exercise more, your blood sugar should decrease, maybe to the point where your doctor will adjust medication levels. Diabetics need control in their lives in order to control blood sugar. Exercise at about the same time each day and following similar eating and medication patterns. A good time is about two hours after meals, when blood sugar is higher. Test blood sugar before and after exercise to avoid problems or a crisis. If your blood sugar is below 100 mg/dl before exercise, consume a snack before starting. Don't exercise if blood sugar is 60 mg/dl or below or you are showing any symptoms of hypoglycemia: double vision, nervousness, trembling, heavy sweating, or clammy skin. Exercise with a partner and avoid exercise in extreme weather conditions. Carry an emergency sugar supply and wear an identification bracelet that indicates you are a diabetic. Diabetics should review all the information about controlling blood sugar throughout the day and consider the impact of exercise. Discuss your exercise plan with a diabetes educator or your doctor.

> *"A journey of a thousand miles begins with but a single step."*
> —LAO TZE (c. 604–521 B.C.), *Tao Te Ching (Book of Changes)*

The First Step: Get Up and Get Moving

Getting started with exercise is as simple as getting up and shutting off the TV. Then move—do something, anything. A study at the Harvard School of Public Health showed that watching television is hazardous to your health. The study compared a group of men who rarely watched television with those watching twenty-one to forty hours per week and those who watch more. The men who watched more than forty hours per week were three times as likely to develop diabetes, and the middle group had two times the risk of those who rarely watched. So, get up and take a walk around the block. Take your children with you, go to the park, or toss a ball back and forth. If you are in a bit better shape, walk a couple of miles, play a bit of baseball, touch football, or basketball. If you have been sedentary, start slowly and talk to your doctor first. You can increase your level of activity by parking a couple of blocks from your office or from some store. Take the stairs instead of the elevator.

Some things you might try to get started include:

- ♦ Set a specific time each day, or every other day, that you will be active.
- ♦ Begin with an easy activity such as walking ten to fifteen minutes during your lunchtime.
- ♦ Try to do some errands or tasks on foot, by walking, rather than take the car.
- ♦ Do some vigorous yard work or scrub the tub or your car.
- ♦ Get off the bus early and walk part of the distance.
- ♦ Instead of a coffee break, take a short walking break.
- ♦ Don't call or e-mail the person down the hall at work; get up and walk over to his or her office.

Aerobic Exercise

There are two basic classifications of physical activities. Both are essential to a fully rounded exercise program. Aerobic activities use the large muscle groups and give the heart and lungs a good workout. Many people think of all aerobics as very high intensity acitivities like running a marathon, cross-country skiing, or "boot camp type" aerobic classes. There are many aerobic activities that can raise your heart rate in the "target zone," but have lower impact or are less strenuous. They include jogging, swimming, cycling, dancing, rowing, or fast walking. Anaerobic exercise uses muscles at high intensity and at a high rate of work for a short period of time. Anaerobic exercise helps increase muscle strength and allows us to be ready for quick bursts of speed. Anaerobic exercise

HEART POINT

Your maximum heart rate is dependent on your physical condition and what medications you are taking. Calcium channel blockers, beta blockers, and other heart medications lower your heart rate and blood pressure. Discuss this with your cardiologist before starting an exercise program.

occurs in sprinting, heavy weight lifting, or any rapid bursts of hard exercise. Many truly anaerobic exercises are not appropriate for heart patients, so be sure to consult your physician. Lower repetitions using lighter weights and stretching exer-cises can safely build strength and flexibility without harm.

Measuring Your Pulse

In order to know if you are within your target range you need to learn to take your pulse. Each time you feel a pulse, it is a heartbeat, and by counting them you can figure out how many times your heart is beating per minute. There are several pulse points on the body, including the wrist, neck, and chest, but the easiest location is the neck. Take two fingertips and move them along the outer edge of your windpipe and press gently until you feel the throb of your heart beating. Watch the second hand of a watch and count all of the beats for a ten-second time period. Multiply that number by six and that will give you your heart rate per minute.

An easier way to know your heart rate is with a pulse watch. This digital watch continuously monitors your heart rate and has stopwatch and other

---

FIGURING YOUR TARGET ZONE

1. Find your maximum heart rate by subtracting your age from 220. (This is an average. Check with your doctor before starting any exercise program as your physical condition, prescription medications, and other factors affect your actual maximum heart rate.)

2. Calculate 60 percent to 85 percent of your maximum heart rate (multiply by .60 and .85).

For a fifty year old, for example, 60 percent to 85 percent of the maximum heart rate is 102 to 144 beats per minute (220−50=170; 170 x .85=144). Fast walking and low-impact aerobics will raise your heart rate to within the low end of the target range, about 60 percent to 75 percent.

---

typical timepiece functions. During exercise, heart patients can always know their heart rate with a quick look at the watch, a specific measure of how intense they are exercising. The stopwatch feature is also helpful in knowing how long you have been exercising.

The Talk Test

There are other simple ways to gauge the intensity of your exercise. The first is called the "talk test." You should be able to talk to a companion throughout your workout. If your breathing is so labored because of the exercise that you cannot talk, slow down until you can. If you have pain during exercise, especially in the chest, neck, jaw, back, throat, or arms, slow down and stop. If the pain does not stop in a few minutes, or after three nitroglycerin tablets, call 911. Pain is your body's way of telling you there is a problem. Do not "work through" pain. Sweating is normal during exercise; however, if you get "chills," slow down or do less.

DARRELL'S STORY

"After experiencing pain in my arms during my health walks through the park, I slowed down and visited my primary care doctor. He said it was some sort of back pain. My wife, suspecting I was loafing, then started telling me I should 'work through' the pain. It is very important to listen to your body and do no more than it is telling you to (even when your wife says so). In spite of a bad diagnosis, that knowledge of my own body helped keep me alive—I did not attempt to 'work through it.'"

Types of Aerobic Exercise

Any exercise that raises your heart rate and keeps it in your target zone is an aerobic exercise. High-intensity activities include cross-country skiing, jogging, swimming, aerobics classes, and playing soccer or basketball. The advantage of any of these choices is that you can burn up more calories and get fit in less time. As we age, our bodies may not be able to take the impact of feet pounding the hard ground and of jolting every joint in our body, or because of other physical challenges we may need to work out at less intense levels. High-impact exercise will be tough on our bodies. Some high-impact activities include running or jogging, basketball, volleyball, jumping, rope skipping, aerobic dancing, and downhill skiing. Low-impact alternatives include walking, hiking, cycling, stationary cycling, swimming, rowing, and cross-country skiing.

A *Lifestyle Walking Plan*

One way to incorporate healthy activity into your day without having a structured exercise program is to add steps. One way to measure how active you are is by counting the number of steps you take per day. Research has shown that inactive people take only 2,000 to 4,000 steps per day, moderately active people take 5,000 to 7,000 steps per day, and active people take over 10,000 steps per day. A simple, low-cost way to count those steps is with a pedometer. Wear it on a belt, about midline on your thigh. The high-end models, about $35, will keep track of all your steps, convert steps into miles walked, and show you calories burned. Just wearing a pedometer will encourage you to move around more and keep track during the day. First, measure how many steps you currently take in an average day. Second, set a goal for a higher number of steps per day. You can easily add more steps and become more active. As you become more active and achieve your first fitness goal, you will be encouraged to move to even higher levels of fitness. If you have been inactive, this is a good beginning. It also is a nice complement to more traditional structured exercise programs.

HEART POINT

DOING STEPS IN THE OFFICE: Purchase a long telephone cord for your receiver. Get up and move around the desk while you are on the telephone. You will be amazed how many extra steps you can add each day.

Health Walking

Perhaps the best, certainly one of the best, exercise programs is walking. Experts are beginning to believe that those power workouts at health clubs may not be the best form of exercise for most people. This seems particularly true for the population most at risk for heart disease and those actively fighting it. High-impact aerobics and running have been popular forms of exercise, but as we age, our joints, specifically knees, don't like any jarring workouts. Walking doesn't harm the joints or have many other negatives.

What we refer to as "health walking" is walking at a fast enough pace to raise your heart rate into your target zone, 60 percent to 75 percent of your maximum heart rate. Ideally, your cardiologist has determined your maximum heart rate during a treadmill stress test. With the doctor's help you will be able to set your target zone for the ideal health walk. For most people, walking at a brisk pace (three to four miles per hour) for thirty minutes, four to five days per week will produce good results. Dr. JoAnn Manson, Chief of Preventive Medicine at Harvard's Brigham and Women's Hospital, suggests if everyone walked that much we could cut chronic diseases 30 percent to 40 percent.

Any good and safe exercise program starts slowly and gradually increases over time. With your doctor's approval, start by walking twelve to fifteen minutes a day. Strive for a target heart range of 40 percent to 60 percent of maximum heart rate. Walk on alternate days for three days per week. Do this for four to six weeks; extend the time if you were really out of shape.

For the second phase, add a few minutes of exercise time every two or three weeks. Work up to exercising continuously for twenty to thirty minutes. Do this from three to five days per week. Stay at this level for about four

HEART POINT

WALKING SHOES: This is your only required equipment; select them carefully. A good pair will cost about $60 to $90 and last about 300 to 500 miles depending on your weight. Go to a quality athletic shoe store with employees who will work to fit you properly. If you wear shoes out in an uneven pattern, describe that to the salesperson. They should know about that specific problem and what shoe will best compensate for it. Some brands are sold in widths to accommodate wide feet. Take the socks you will be wearing while walking to try on shoes.

months, longer if you are straining. During this phase, your target heart rate should be 50 percent to 75 percent of maximum.

The third phase is to exercise from three to five days per week, for thirty to sixty minutes each day, at a target heart rate of 60 percent to 75 percent of your maximum. At that level you are getting considerable health benefits from your efforts and have cut your risk of disease considerably.

Good Walking Form

To avoid injury and get the most from your exercise you should maintain good walking form. Most people slouch and hunch their shoulders. You want to keep your back straight (think of stretching out your spine) and eyes forward, not down toward the ground. To speed up, take faster steps rather than trying to stretch your stride—it should be natural, never forced. A natural walking stride means pushing off with your toes and landing on your heel. Keep your elbows bent about ninety degrees and move your arms in cadence with your pace. This will give you a more complete workout. Do not use weights; they can lead to injury. To increase the intensity of your workout (after you are in good shape), walk in a hilly location. Think back to being on a treadmill and increasing the grade. Even a slight incline will increase the amount of work you must do.

Gardening for the Heart of It

Gardening is another wonderful activity that gets you moving. A major advantage is that for many people it doesn't even seem like exercise—they love doing it. Darrell has been gardening for many years. He became so involved with gardening that he changed careers, worked in horticulture, and became a garden writer. Gardening is an activity that promotes good health for everybody. The physical component seems obvious. It is necessary to do some physical activity on a regular basis, so why not something you enjoy. Raking leaves or hoeing utilizes 5 to 6 calories per minute, the same as cycling at eight miles per hour. Digging in the garden equates to cycling at ten miles per hour and burns 6 to 7 calories per minute. These are preferable to riding on a lawn mower and burning only 2 to 4 calories an hour, though that is a bit more than watching television. Using an old-fashioned reel-type push mower burns even more calories. If you are shoveling topsoil and mulch or cutting down trees, you will get an aerobic workout. Digging and raking use the same energy as volleyball or brisk walking. Shoveling, chopping wood, and mowing with a push mower is as much work as doubles tennis, fencing, or downhill skiing.

Every bit of exercise helps the body become and stay healthy. Gardening is one of the activities that is a healthy lifestyle habit. If you garden at least thirty minutes a day you will decrease your risk of heart disease and other chronic diseases. Gardening improves strength, flexibility, and endurance. Heavy gardening work, such as digging and chopping wood, builds upper body strength. Reaching out to pull weeds or to push soil around new transplants stretches muscles and improves flexibility. Working in the garden for several hours for several days will add to your endurance. It's certainly better to spread your work out so you work from thirty minutes to a few hours each day, rather than work six or eight hours on Saturday. The latter is a sure way to end up with very sore muscles and a negative view of gardening. It's like any other physical activity, you need to start slow and add more hours over time.

Have you ever seen a really fat gardener? Not too many anyway. Research tells us that age is no barrier to exercise, and the more you do and the more years you do it, the better off you will be. Darrell's great-grandmother, who lived to be ninety-five, maintained her cottage garden until her death. Even as a young child he knew how important her garden was to her. Other famous gardeners who lived long, productive lives include Adelma Simmons, Ruth Stout, and Harold Epstein.

Gardening also improves mental attitude. Although harder to measure, research has confirmed that the mind–body connection exists. Most will agree that a positive mental attitude is beneficial in overcoming disease. Harvard-educated, natural medicine guru Dr. Andrew Weil says that we all need to connect with nature. He suggests that we have flowers around us all of the time. He takes pleasure in many forms of gardening including growing bulbs, cactus, and other unusual plants inside his house and in his garden. He, like many others, takes great comfort in the reminders of being part of the natural world. He also suggests that the way to eat more fresh fruit and vegetables without consuming poisons is to grow some or most of your own food and describes the satisfaction of harvesting your own crops while working off daily stress.

Gardening is a healthy activity on many levels. Dr. Bruno Cortis, author of *Heart & Soul,* suggests that gardening is ideal for cardiac patients. It is totally absorbing, allowing you to forget your problems, and it usually takes place outdoors, where you breathe fresh air. You are more in touch with nature. Dr. Cortis also says that houseplants help to calm people and make them more optimistic. He points out a study that found that hospital patients whose rooms faced a garden recovered more quickly than those with rooms facing a wall. (Darrell's room at Mt. Sinai Hospital faced a large atrium full of plants!)

This is only a sampling of the evidence that gardening is a health-promoting activity. Truthfully, we knew it already—those of us who garden, anyway. We feel better after working, or even just walking, in our gardens. So, this is a reminder to do just that: stop and smell the gardenias, violets, lavender, or even roses, if that's your preference. Invite someone else, particularly someone who is ill or has been feeling down, to enjoy the garden with you. Maybe take part of the garden to them by cutting some flowers or taking a houseplant to someone who can use the boost. Share the joy!

Warm Up, Stretch, and Cool Down

It's a good idea to warm up before doing any strenuous activity. A few minutes of brisk walking will get you started and prepare your body for more. If you are health walking at a fast pace, start out at a slower speed for several minutes. Stretching before and after your exercise can avoid strained muscles. Give yourself five to ten minutes to cool down.

Keep a Record

You should record the amount of exercise you do each day. You can also record all of your walking if you use a pedometer. As your minutes of exercise become hours, and your miles add up, you will get a sense of accomplishment. You will see your progress written down. It will also give you an idea of your level of fit-

EXERCISE LOG

Date	Exercise Type	Duration	Target Heart Rate	How You Felt

ness. We have provided a sample Exercise Log. Record the date, type of exercise, duration, target heart rate, and how you felt on your Exercise Log sheet.

Motivation: Keeping at It

"The first step is one which makes the rest of our days."
—VOLTAIRE (1694–1778)

We realize that it may be difficult to start and maintain an exercise program. While there may be no perfect solution to the problem, improving and maintaining a healthy lifestyle is paramount to *Surviving with Heart.* It helps to break major projects or goals into small steps. If you start to waver in your resolve, think about the Lewis and Clark Expedition moving across America. It took them years, on foot, to travel from the East Coast to the West Coast, facing uncountable hurdles along the way. They achieved their goal through perseverance. A frequently noted entry in their journals simply stated, "We continued on." That's what you need to do: take small steps each day toward fitness and a healthy lifestyle. You did not become overweight, out of shape, and with clogged arteries overnight. It took years, so don't think you will solve your problems in a few weeks or even months. Here are some suggestions to help you "continue on."

♦ Start slow and do not expect instant results. It takes months to reach major goals. Remember that every bit of progress improves your health and will soon lower your risk of a heart attack.

♦ Set numerical goals. Don't have a goal of "I'm going to exercise more." Set specific goals such as, "In one year I will walk forty-five minutes at a four-miles-per-hour pace on four days each week."

♦ Break your goals into attainable steps for your health and fitness level. Example: Goal 1: Walk fifteen minutes per day three days per week for four weeks. Goal 2: Add three minutes per day (total, eighteen minutes) for next four weeks. Goal 3: Add three minutes per day (total, twenty-one minutes) for next four weeks. Keep going like that until you reach your one-year goal. It's important to work through the six-month mark, which is a stumbling point for many.

♦ Exercise with a friend or caregiver. With both of you committed, it is much harder to just skip exercise. You don't want to disappoint the other person.

♦ Set a regular time for exercise. Once exercise becomes a regular part of your life it is no longer an intrusion. It is a time commitment, but remember, it is helping you feel and look better and extending your life.

♦ Keep an exercise log. Recording what you do every day will reinforce your positive feelings about exercise and what you are doing.

♦ Have your doctor ask to see your exercise log (and food diary) at each visit. It gets her involved, and you will have a significant person to share your accomplishments with and motivate you.

♦ Recruit friends and family to join your healthy lifestyle. This is important for family members who you know are at risk for heart disease. Even if they are not close enough to exercise with on a regular basis, you can reinforce each other's efforts.

♦ If you have a setback or relapse into less healthy habits, start over. Many people do not succeed the first, or second, or even third time they attempt a healthier lifestyle, but *do not give up.* These are setbacks, not failures. The only failure is not trying.

♦ Reward yourself for achieving specific goals, but not with a large, rich meal in a restaurant. Buy of a new outfit for your slimmer, healthier body, or a weekend at a spa, a special book, or a boxed set of CDs by a favorite artist.

♦ Enjoy the new, toned, healthier you!

GET INTO CARDIAC REHABILITATION

Historic Heart Patient Treatment

If you had a heart attack in the 1920s to 1940s, your doctor would likely have ordered you to bed rest for six weeks in the hospital. After discharge, your doctor would likely advise "limited activity." Between 1940 and 1950 "chair treatment" was introduced. A nurse helped the patient move from bed to a chair and then back again. By the 1960s, research results proved that an active patient recovered faster and better than resting ones, and in-hospital rehabilitation began. With increasing medical costs in the 1980s and 1990s, insurance coverage shifted from in-hospital to outpatient cardiac rehabcenters.

DARRELL'S STORY

"I started walking again immediately after my surgery. The day after the surgery the nurses encouraged me to walk around in the hospital. I got out of bed, with help the first time, and started walking. I figure I walked about a mile that day (there were measured distances marked with hearts on the floor of the hospital), then again the next day. I started walking regularly the day after I got home from the hospital. In a short time, I was walking several miles per day every day and kept pushing my cardiologist to let me walk faster and raise my heart rate into an aerobic target range. My cardiologist joked that by the time my rehab started, thirty days after surgery for me, I wouldn't need it. Rehab helped me safely work to higher intensity levels and get into even better shape. There were lectures, handouts, and encouragement from the staff, along with a special camaraderie with my fellow rehab patients. Other patients needed to learn that exercise was not only safe, but also necessary, for good health. I also learned that patients who continued with rehab and exercise avoided future problems."

In the past, cardiac rehabilitation programs were directed only to heart attack survivors. Today, virtually all heart patients can and should be referred to rehabilitation centers. Bypass surgery, angioplasty, valve replacements, and even heart transplant patients benefit from rehab. Rehab is suited for someone with multiple risk factors. Insurance companies would be well advised to get at-risk patients into rehabilitation, saving them the high cost of cardiac surgery in the future.

How Does Cardiac Rehab Work?

Cardiac rehab is composed of two major components: exercise training plus education and counseling. Exercise training teaches the patient to exercise safely, improve stamina, and strengthen muscles. A staff member creates an exercise plan based on your physical ability and needs.

The education and counseling helps you understand your heart problems and what you can do to reduce your risks in the future. The cardiac rehab team, including doctors, nurses, exercise specialists, physical and occupational therapists, dietitians, and psychologists or other behavior therapists, teaches you how to cope with the stress of heart disease and adjust to a new lifestyle.

There are over 500 cardiac rehab centers throughout America, most affiliated with a hospital or with a significant cardiac center. Most cardiac rehab takes place in a group setting with individualized patient plans. There are some home-based rehab plans where you are connected to an EKG machine and monitored by telephone as you exercise. At first glance, a rehab center looks much like a health club, though with an older clientele and few young, hard-body types.

How Safe Is Rehab?

Cardiac rehab is one of the safest ways and places for a heart patient to exercise. There are always trained medical professionals on staff there while you are exercising. Throughout the workout, personnel monitor patients constantly with telemetry heart monitors and regular blood pressure readings. Patients also monitor their own pulse throughout their workout. A significant goal of rehab is to teach you how to exercise safely as vigorously as you can.

What Will Cardiac Rehab Do for Me?

The professional staff will set specific goals for each patient depending on need and physical abilities. All programs work to reduce symptoms and risk factors for heart disease and to avoid additional heart problems. Rehab teaches you to:

- Exercise safely, increase fitness level, and improve muscle tone, which improves energy level and attitude. It helps strengthen your heart and body and gets you back to activities sooner.
- Understand nutrition, healthy food consumption, ideal body weight, and weight control techniques that will help you improve blood pressure, blood glucose, and lipid control, which make you feel better and have more energy.
- Quit smoking, which lowers risk of heart attack and other blood vessel problems. It also decreases your risk of asthma, bronchitis, emphysema, and a number of cancers and leads to better health for you and your loved ones.
- Manage stress better so you can better contend with life's problems, including your illness.
- Deal with the mild depression that often follows a heart attack or surgery by getting to know others with similar challenges along with providing professional help. If you are seriously depressed, get additional professional help.

Selecting a Rehab Center

You should select your rehab center carefully. Determine what centers are in your area by checking with your medical team, insurance provider, and the Yellow Pages. Visit all of the centers in your area; ask for a tour and talk to staff and patients. Consider how much time it takes to get to the center—you will be going there three times per week for about twelve weeks or more. Think about traffic and parking at the time of day you will be attending (try to schedule your visit for that time of day so you really know). Investigate what services are included in the rehab "package" and other optional services you might need. Low-fat cooking, stress and anger management, and stop-smoking classes may be offered at an additional charge. What are the costs, and what does your insurance company cover? Many insurance providers will pay for a six- to twelve-week "Phase II" program. You may want to continue—and research shows it is beneficial—for additional weeks beyond the basic program.

DARRELL'S STORY

"All cardiac rehab programs are not the same. I did not have a good experience with the first center that I was referred to by my cardiologist. It is only a few minutes from my house and seemed a logical choice. On my first visit to register, I found the center understaffed and some seemed unprofessional. I complained about the handling and got an unsatisfactory response. I wrote a letter to my cardiologist, with a copy to the center, explained the situation, and asked him to refer me to another center. (If you have any problems with referrals, centers, or doctors, tell your doctor about it.) I called St. Francis Hospital's Cardiac Fitness and Rehabilitation Center, made an appointment, and visited. The center was an additional thirty minutes from my home. The extra time was worth it because of the quality of staff and services. Select your rehab center, and all medical services, carefully."

BE A HEART CARE PARTNER

JACK'S STORY
(heart patient, 72)

"My wife has been my main support. We work as a team together to stay fit and in good health physically, mentally, and spiritually. We try to have as little stress as possible. We travel and read and are active in events that include friends who have a lot of the same interests as we do."

WHEN A FRIEND or loved one is diagnosed with heart disease, it should be a wake-up call for the caregiver. If the heart patient lives with the caregiver, it is almost impossible for him to successfully manage a lifestyle reversal if his caregiver is not following the same or a similar plan. Both patient and caregiver should be following a reversal plan that includes a heart-smart diet, regular exercise, and stress reduction. Working together at maintaining a healthy lifestyle holds the patient and the caregiver accountable to each other. The patient will not feel like the only one making sacrifices. Plus, lots of things are more fun if you do them with someone you enjoy being around. How can you encourage each other?

- Sit down together and set small, attainable goals and stick with them. Decide where you need to make individual and joint changes in each area: diet, exercise, and stress reduction.
- Encourage each other to be "good" even when you are not together. Call regularly just to ask, "What did you have for lunch?" "What was your blood sugar this morning?" or "Tell me how many vegetables you had yesterday."
- Send motivational e-mails and cards to each other.
- Put inspirational messages or notes around the house; the refrigerator door or bathroom mirror are effective places.
- Stick notes in lunch bags to encourage good eating habits.
- Exercise together. Walk in the park, the mall, the neighborhood, on the school track, or at your cardiac rehab program. Agree to park a distance away from the entrance to the supermarket or mall. Challenge each other to see who can walk the most miles in a month.
- Go to the grocery store together. Plan healthy menus and help each other get only the needed ingredients.
- Put allowed snacks in clear plastic bags so it is obvious how many are left! It makes it harder to "cheat."
- Refuse to add stress to each other's lives. Adopt a lifestyle that is as stress-free as possible. Plan your trips and outings as low-stress experiences that you can both enjoy.
- Help each other find individual outlets that help you relax. Reduce how much time you spend on the road.

ELLEN'S STORY

"When my dad began having heart problems, I started learning all I could in order to help him. After I found out how at risk I was, I started changing my lifestyle. I knew I could not preach to him about a healthy lifestyle

if I was not practicing one. We have even challenged each other at different times to lose five or ten pounds in order to stay on track. My mother
tries to find great healthy recipes and really watches Dad's sugar and salt
intake. We enjoy swapping new 'healthy
finds' with each other. It makes me feel like
I am a part of their efforts to live a healthy
life and it keeps me 'on the wagon.' Several
patients have confidentially told us that it
has been hard to change their lifestyle
habits when the person they live with has not."

> "Set small, attainable
> goals and stick with
> them."

Assess Your Risk Factors

Any exercise program or diet product recommends that you see your doctor
before beginning. That's a great idea! Just as the patient should know the
healthy range for all his or her vital signs, so should any caregiver. We all need
to know the healthy range for our weight, blood pressure, heart rate, blood
sugar, and cholesterol. Not only will it help you feel in charge of your health,
but it will help you identify more with what your patient is facing. If you have
heart disease in your family history, be sure to tell the doctor. Complete a
family health history (see Star Point One) to take with you to the doctor.

A 1994 survey by the Centers for Disease Control and Prevention found
that 80 percent of adult Americans have at least one condition or habit that
could put them at risk for heart disease. See where you fit in. Check any of the
following that apply:

Checklists
Major Risk Factors

_____ 1. My immediate family member (mother, father, brother, or sister)
has had heart disease.

_____ 2. My immediate family member had a heart attack before
age fifty.

_____ 3. I am a smoker.

    4. I have high blood pressure (pressure above 140/90 mm Hg)

    5. I have total blood cholesterol above 240 mg/dl.

    6. I am at least twenty pounds (or more) overweight.

    7. I have diabetes or one of my immediate family members has diabetes.

Secondary Risk Factors

    8. I rarely exercise.

    9. I am a postmenopausal woman and not on hormone replacement.

   10. I take oral contraceptives.

   11. I often eat red meat, full-fat dairy products, fast food, fatty desserts, and snack foods.

   12. I eat fewer than six daily servings of grains, five servings of vegetables, and two servings of fruit.

   13. I use addictive drugs.

   14. I am a heavy drinker (more than two drinks per day).

If you checked one or more of the Major Risk Factors listed, you could be at an increased risk of developing heart disease. In addition, if you checked one or more of the Secondary Risk Factors, your lifestyle is putting you even more at risk, and you need to start making immediate changes.

MARLA'S STORY
(caregiver, 51)

"After my mom saw the cardiologist, it made me start thinking more about my own health. I finally went to the doctor and found out my blood pressure was dangerously high. I've tried several medications now and even switched doctors to make sure I am getting the best help and information. I have started losing weight and I'm trying to exercise more. I am doing for myself exactly what I have been telling my mother to do."

Celebrate Success

Dealing with heart disease and all the patient–caregiver dynamics will take a toll on you if you do not take the time to find the "good stuff." Look for the positive—the silver linings. Celebrate anything and everything. Obviously, we don't recommend that you indulge in celebrations that undermine your healthy lifestyle, but we do encourage you to find ways to acknowledge large and small milestones. For example:

♦ When a weight-loss goal is achieved
♦ When blood sugar or blood pressure readings stay at a desired level for a week or more
♦ After a positive medical checkup
♦ For a surgery anniversary
♦ When a medication is discontinued because a patient's physical report is so good
♦ When you go a whole week without getting angry or stressed out

Celebrations can include sending a card or e-mail, having friends over for dinner, taking a trip, buying something special (special but not chocolate!), purchasing new clothes, calling extended family or friends, or sending flowers or balloons.

ELLEN'S STORY

"When I put important dates on a new calendar each year, in addition to birthdays, I include surgery anniversaries. I mark down my dad's, Darrell's, and others. They are special people, and we are all blessed that they were given a second chance. It's worth remembering them and their lives each year. I send a card or simply say, 'Happy anniversary' in a phone call."

STAR POINT SIX

Embrace Support

"It is not so much our friends' help that helps us as the confident knowledge that they will help us."

—EPICURUS (341–270 B.C.)

RELATIONSHIPS PLAY A significant role in recovery. Patients, caregivers, and others interact in powerful ways. We show you some benefits of this support for patients and caregivers. We give you ways to increase all types of support and to utilize the connection between the mind and body.

ACCEPTING PHYSICAL SUPPORT

WE WANT TO stress that *if friends offer to help out, let them!* Usually when friends ask if they can help, they sincerely want to assist. Do not assume that they think you cannot handle everything. Many caregivers admit that they have a major tendency to do too much. Some patients try to do too much too soon. If you are the "too busy" type, be careful. Try to identify what makes you give in to the tendency. Some caregivers admit to doing too much to indirectly get attention because so much of their time and attention goes to the patient. Both patients and caregivers need to monitor feelings of fatigue. If you are consistently overwhelmed, we suggest you consider the following tips:

- If finances allow, get some assistance—help for the patient or with yard and house maintenance. Save the "back-breaking" tasks for someone who can easily handle them. Be very specific about what you need someone to do.
- Allow friends to drive you to the doctor.
- Accept meals from friends and family.
- Let others who volunteer run errands for you to the grocery store or pharmacy.
- If you have children or grandchildren, involve them in smaller tasks that will help them feel a part of the caregiving process.

There is another side to physical support. Rehab centers provide great opportunities for patients to resume physical exercise while being monitored, but sometimes caregivers need to "get more physical" too. Find a neighborhood group to go walking with. Join a health club and sign up for specific exercise classes, such as water aerobics, so you can get your workout and feel supported at the same time.

DARRELL'S STORY

"The outpouring of support was almost overwhelming. Some people prayed for me, and others hosted group meditations—all of it made me feel wonderful. Support came from far and wide, sometimes from surprising sources and in unexpected ways. Even though my recovery was amazingly fast, that outpouring of support and caring had a huge, long-lasting effect of me."

MAXIMIZING SOCIAL SUPPORT

HEART PATIENTS, AND all others facing major illness or physical challenge, must look for ways to maximize their social support. Very few people have large nuclear families nearby anymore. Families are smaller, and members are scattered far and wide. When you are hospitalized in an emergency, or for surgery, people seem to know exactly what to do and how to behave. They come to the hospital to visit or send cards and flowers. But once you go home, they may not know your needs.

At home, your problems are different. You are there alone or with a small core of family. Your life is not the same as before. You are out of work, you have less energy, you may be fearful, recreation patterns are disrupted, and you may have financial pressures. How do you increase your social support under those conditions?

Start by figuring out who in your wide network of friends and organizations can and will provide support. Create a list of all of those people, including those who only would be willing or able to help in a very limited way. The length of the list will give you comfort. Next, start to analyze the variables of the type of support each individual or organization can provide. What are their current commitments? Do they have family or career obligations that will limit their ability to help? Do they live a great distance away?

You now have defined who is able to provide specific types of help and support. For instance, there is a group of neighbors, with cars, who are willing and able to shop for groceries for you. Set up a schedule and rotate those helpers as needed. Let some friends who are far away know how much you would appreciate telephone calls and e-mails for the time you are home-bound. Let colleagues at work know that you would like to stay up to date on office politics and the status of work projects. Select only the positive from work: contact the people you like and ask about projects you feel positive about. Let some of your nieces know that it would be nice to see them on the second or fourth weekends of the month and your grandchildren on the first and third weekends. Figure out for others on the list how they can help in ways that fit with their lives and present commitments. This will increase your social contacts. Avoid negative people and situations—this is about moving forward and feeling good.

CATHY'S STORY

(potential heart patient, 52)

Cathy is a garden writer friend of Darrell's who lives halfway across the country from him. She supported him during his surgeries and problems. When she found out that she needed to have an angiogram, she let friends all over the United States know about it. Darrell called her and talked about his experiences. He also sent Cathy e-mails and told her to call any-time with any questions and assured her that he would help any way he could. After Cathy's angiogram, she sent this e-mail to a number of her friends:

"I was overwhelmed by the outpouring of kind wishes and positive thoughts . . . and they worked. According to the surgeon, my heart and its arteries are enviable—in perfect condition! The test itself went very smoothly and I was able to watch the entire procedure (they even gave me a printout to 'put on your refrigerator.' It looks like a black-and-white illustration from an anatomy text). Thanks so much for your kind thoughts. Sometimes it takes a serious scare like this to make you appreci-ate how many great friends you have. And I am truly grateful for every one."

In this story, Darrell's friend Cathy didn't have heart disease, but she did have a good support system. She reached out across the country to tap it, and her friends responded. You can do the same.

Look for formal support sources to add to all of your personal contacts. Look for organizations, self-help groups, or social service agencies. Ask for referrals from your hospital, doctors, friends, and religious organizations.

Support Networks Save Lives

When Darrell was going through heart surgery and recovery, he was aware of feeling better because of support from family, friends, organizations, and gar-den writer contacts. There is more to it than just "good feelings." Research has shown that patients with a good social support system in place recover more quickly and live longer. Divorced, separated, single, or widowed people are more likely to die than those who are married, even if it's not a particularly good marriage. Those individuals without strong social connections are more likely to have heart disease, cancer, depression, arthritis, or pregnancy problems. Patients shouldn't "tough it out" alone but embrace the love, help, and support from others and seek out more.

It would seem to make sense that "loners" would have greater difficulty dealing with virtually any major life crisis. After heart surgery, the simple physical reality of not having someone to drive you, or help lift things (no lifting of more than a few pounds for several weeks after surgery), or grocery shop for you would add stress. Many people would have trouble following doctor's orders under those circumstances. A patient may try to do too much and damage surgical stitching or do other damage to the body by exceeding the doctor's restrictions. What about the mind? Does your attitude change with support?

It is more complicated than simple physical needs and dangers. Researchers have investigated the link between social factors and health. There are many types of social support, from close family and friends to work relationships with your coworkers and boss, to more casual contacts with members of clubs and religious organizations. All are valuable and are a positive force in healing and life.

In Alameda County, California, in the 1960s, researchers looked at over 5,000 people and the links between their health and social factors. Results showed clearly that those individuals who were the least socially integrated (having the fewest relationships—contacts with friends, relatives, spouse, churches, and clubs) had the greatest risk of dying prematurely. Results of that study were more recently revalidated in Dr. Lisa F. Berkman and Dr. Lester Breslow's book *Health and Ways of Living: The Alameda County Study*. A larger Swedish study of 17,433 women and men had a similar conclusion. Those with the fewest relationships and social contacts had a death rate 50 percent higher than those with the highest number of contacts. These studies and others show that results apply equally for men and women, rich or poor, and all races.

Building Your Support System

You and your caregiver need to list activities that will require extra assistance. If you are going to require some help at home for a while, ask the hospital discharge planner or patient representative to give you the names of local organizations that provide nursing, home care, companionship, housekeeping, and other services. Knowing where to call if you need assistance will keep you from worrying.

Mended Hearts, Brave Hearts, and More

Mended Hearts is a national organization, with ties to the American Heart Association, that supports individuals with heart problems, their families, and caregivers. Their members speak from the experience of someone with heart disease. They have trained members who talk to people immediately after a diagnosis of heart disease, when a patient is scheduled for surgery, after surgery in the hospital, or after returning home. They talk to patients, family members, and caregivers. There are currently over 250 chapters, most in the United States and a few in Canada. There is also a new program to help people via the Internet. Therefore, even if you are not near one of the chapters, help is available. Make this organization part of your support plan.

DARRELL'S STORY

"After my bypass surgery, I recovered so quickly that I almost missed my visit from a Brave Hearts of St. Francis Hospital volunteer. They give each heart patient a heart-shaped pillow. You can hold that pillow against your chest and your 'zipper,' that long surgery scar down your chest, when you feel a cough approaching. That will help avoid a painful moment or damaging your stitching. I think the 'hugging' action is also practical and makes you feel better. The support organization newsletters often print a coupon good for 'one hug.' Make up a sheet of hug coupons for your patient."

There are also other local, or hospital-specific, heart organizations, such as Brave Hearts, at some other hospitals throughout the United States. Brave Hearts and Mended Hearts members contacted Darrell during and after his surgery. He is a member of both groups and supports their efforts and goals. These groups also have meetings, heart-education lectures, and social events. (See Resources for contact information.)

Reach Out and Help Someone

When you are back on your feet, remember to return the favor for someone else in need. One of Darrell's gardening friends fell down an unprotected flight of stairs during house remodeling and broke her clavicle. After returning from the hospital, Sara Jane was unable to leave her house or do a number of otherwise normal tasks for weeks. She said, "I will never forget my friends. They have called, shopped for me, cooked for me, and one even helped me bathe!" She will remember. Even as you recuperate, you can reach out to others by calling them, sending cards, notes, and e-mail.

We know the personal satisfaction of helping others. Some researchers suggest that helping others is another form of social attachment that releases endorphins, which create the typical feel-good "runner's high." It now seems that helping others is also good for our health. Henry Dreher, in his book *The Immune Power Personality,* describes how volunteers, in self-assessment surveys, describe themselves as healthier than others their own age. Measures of the volunteers' absolute health showed that they were correct. The more they helped others the higher their self-assessments of their health. Those positive feelings continue long after the actual volunteer work is finished.

Relate to Rehab

Many cardiac rehabilitation programs offer helpful assistance for caregivers and patients. Plugging into these opportunities strengthens the patient–caregiver bond and allows you to get to know other people facing similar situations. We encourage caregivers to call the rehab program their patient will attend or presently attends to see if the following is available for you to use:

- ♦ Access to exercise equipment and walking track
- ♦ Caregiver support groups
- ♦ Informational programs for caregivers and patients

JAY'S STORY
(heart patient, 66)

"At first, I wasn't going to try rehab, but a representative visited us in the hospital and made a big spiel. I felt guilty enough that I tried it. I had no energy at first, but getting there and then working out made all the difference. I had not been an exercise person before rehab and now I have my own treadmill at home and exercise regularly."

Seeing a caregiver involved in the rehab program stimulates a patient to stick with it and make progress. Caregivers are empowered by caring professionals who understand how vital their relationship is to the patient's continued recovery. Cardiac rehab offers a safe environment to increase physical activity and resume a normal lifestyle. It can be a wonderful, healthy outlet for both the patient and the caregiver. To learn more about cardiac rehabilitation programs, see the cardiac rehab information in Star Point Five.

ELAINE'S STORY
(caregiver, 65)

"I was so concerned that my husband didn't get his strength back. I almost had to drag him to rehab the first time or two, but then he was ready to go after that. The hospital where he goes lets spouses or caregivers come and exercise also and has special programs just for us. I have met so many other caregivers, and we offer support for each other. They have become like family to us."

ACCEPTING EMOTIONAL SUPPORT

BETSY'S STORY
(caregiver, 74)

"When my husband had surgery I had to take care of everything. Friends came, helped, and stayed. I could not have done it without friends, and they continue to be there for us."

PHYSICAL SUPPORT is helpful, but most often it is the emotional challenges that overwhelm you the most. Simply getting out of the house or taking a walk can help. If you continue to find regular emotional support, you are less likely to become overwhelmed. The following are good for patient and caregiver:

- ♦ Call a friend or relative. Enlist friends you can call when you need to vent. In addition, set up weekly times to routinely call a special friend or family member with whom you can be totally honest about how you feel. Have an understanding that you can cry, cuss, or complain if that is what it takes to help you get through the challenges and feel stronger. Make notes during the week about what you want to say to this person.

- ♦ If you enjoy using the computer, e-mail family and friends regularly. Getting and receiving e-mail can brighten a tough week.

- ♦ Use the computer or a notebook to write to friends and to journal your own thoughts and feelings. Writing helps you get in touch with what you are experiencing and helps you clarify how to get in control of challenging situations.

- ♦ Find other patients and caregivers with whom you can share. Be aware of coworkers, church members, or neighbors who have been touched by heart disease. Hearing the stories of others will let you know that you are not alone.

ACCEPTING INTEGRAL SUPPORT

Mind and Body Team

We know the importance of physical and emotional support, but the importance of the mind–body connection is less well known, though integral to our well-being. The existence of the mind–body connection was questioned and was controversial in the recent past. Most authorities would now agree that there are specific and provable links. A new field of study, psychoneuroimmunology, has evolved. It investigates the connections between the immune system, mind, and nervous system. The research is showing that our feelings and emotions are not just in our minds, but throughout our bodies, and they affect our bodies. We know that our bodies heal minor cuts and problems without a doctor's help. The body somehow knows to stop the blood flow to the cut and seal if off. A few weeks later, the cut is gone. Our body and mind have solved the problem.

Our mind affects all of our defenses and healing. It has a significant impact on all of our battles with disease. Earlier in this book we looked at the negative impact of stress on the body and its link to heart disease. We know that stress is inevitable. We learned in Star Point Five how to counteract stress (and avoid some). While the stress reduction techniques we suggested do counter the negative impact of stress, they can go even further and become a positive force in all our lives. The activities, including deep breathing, exercise, prayer, and meditation put us in control and can transcend simple stress reduction and move us toward wellness. Choosing to be happy and an optimist can be transporting, moving our thoughts and feelings from negative to positive. Making these choices will utilize the mind and body connection to improve your life and overall health. Those choices will also make it easier to "stay on track" with the lifestyle changes in Star Point Five, which helps you fight heart disease.

Pets and Plants

Most of us know the benefits of pets. Millions of us care for cats, dogs, birds, fish, and even snakes. We don't focus on the negatives, the possible dog bites, fleas, allergic reactions, or the mess. We crave the unconditional love of the loyal and nonjudgmental companion. We are reminded of the talk show admonition to find a mate who loves pets.

Pets have a significant positive influence on our health. Heart attack patients have a better chance of survival if they own a pet. One year after their attacks, pet owners had only one-fifth the odds of dying as those without pets. Other research shows that simply petting a cat or dog lowers blood pressure. Watching fish swim around in an aquarium produces a similar result.

The mechanism for these positive changes really isn't known. Some think it is simply that we can take our minds off problems and life's worries. The gentle stroking of a pet can calm and relax us, relieving anxiety. Pets give us a purpose and a reason to smile. We enjoy playful interaction with them. We laugh at their antics. Taking care of pets is nurturing and loving. Even if people are alone they aren't lonely if they have a pet. They are always there through the difficulties of day-to-day life.

Taking care of plants and gardens seems to promote the same type of feelings. Whether it is the connection with nature, an entity so much bigger than ourselves, or that we focus outside our personal needs, we simply feel better. There is the nurturing act of growing something from a seed or cutting. And there is the feel-good satisfaction of giving from your garden—flowers to someone ill or organic vegetables to a friend. The Garden Writers Association of America directs the Plant a Row for the Hungry Program, in which individual gardeners and groups grow vegetables, "in an extra row," for those in need. Gardeners now grow and donate over 1 million pounds of produce every year to worthy organizations—what a great feeling that creates.

Laughter

> "No man is happy who does not think himself so."
>
> —PUBLIUS SYRUS, *Maxim* (584)

We recall a woman who took her doctor a humorous birthday card, on his birthday, during one of her weekly visits for chemotherapy. The next week, he wanted to know where his card was, so she began taking him one each visit. When the series of treatments ended, she was grateful for the thirty minutes each week spent reading, laughing, and selecting that humorous card. He had made her laugh.

You can laugh away stress. Maybe that is a partial explanation of why there is a link between longevity and sense of humor. Raymond A. Moody, Jr., M.D., author of *Laugh after Laugh: The Healing Power of Humor*, suggests that there are connections between the physiological states of the body and humor. Others have pointed out that laughter helps us put things in perspective and break negative thought patterns. Laughter releases chemicals, including endorphins, that are natural painkillers and mood enhancers.

Norman Cousins, in his famous book *Anatomy of an Illness*, suggests that humor and laughter help us block the despair and panic that follow major illness. They also help set the stage for healing. Cousins had cancer and a heart attack and used humorous movies to elevate his mood.

What if you don't feel happy? Fake it. If you decide to be a positive, fun-loving, and hopeful person, that is what you will become. Try this—just start laughing. Maybe try it in front of a mirror when you are home alone and later, move on to small groups of people. Ever notice how infectious laughter is? If you are in a gathering where someone is happy, joyous, and laughs a lot, the mood of the whole group improves. Think of a friend with an unusual or penetrating laugh and the times that you heard it and started feeling better. Associate with people who have fun and laugh a lot, or better yet, become one of them. Someone suggested that the average person laughs fifteen times each day. Commit to laughing more than the average fifteen times each day.

Reaching out and helping others is another way to make you feel better. Turning our attention away from ourselves to someone else or a larger cause does make us feel better. Look for funny cards that you can send to friends who may need a lift. Or, send a cartoon that will make a friend laugh, or e-mail that friend a joke, funny true story, or quote.

The Exceptional Patient

Dr. Bernie Siegel first described the "exceptional patient" in *Love, Medicine & Miracles.* He pointed out common characteristics of these survivors. Dr. Siegel built on the work of psychologist Al Siebert, who studied survivors of a major Korean War battle. The survivors of illness and battle share many traits.

> "Exceptional patients retain control of their lives, especially during a major medical challenge."

Survivors tend to be inner-directed and have a high degree of self-respect and self-acceptance. They approach life with emotional honesty. They use their own standards, rather than others' beliefs, to make choices in life or their health care. They do not allow what others think of them to guide them. This is a core belief; exceptional patients retain control of their lives, especially during a major medical challenge.

Cardiologist Dr. Bruno Cortis, in *Heart & Soul: A Psychological and Spiritual Guide to Preventing and Healing Heart Disease,* says that one responsibility of being a successful patient is looking after your best interests, to get second opinions, to ask questions, and to ask even more questions. It is your health, and you need to lead your health team and be a full participant in your care and do everything you can to get well. This extends to following doctors' instructions, making lifestyle improvements, and taking medicine as prescribed. You are the only person who can improve your lifestyle.

> "You are the only person who can improve your lifestyle."

He suggests that exceptional patients have the same surprise of diagnosis as do all patients, but their response is quite different. They look on the disease as a challenge and, ultimately, a positive way to change their lives. Exceptional patients have hope for the future and the perseverance to change in necessary ways.

Greg Anderson, in *The 22 (Non-Negotiable) Laws of Wellness,* discusses personal accountability. He suggests that rather than our genes and doctors, we have to be in charge of our wellness. There are lifestyle choices that will improve our chances or make our disease worse; we have to choose. We know, or should find out, which behaviors are the most harmful. You should choose to control blood sugar, blood pressure, weight, and stress. If you don't, you will not live as long. *It is your choice.* He goes beyond the physical and suggests that we can choose our emotional and spiritual responses to our challenge. If we allow negative, angry, fearful, or high-stress responses to take over our response to disease and life, we will produce a toxic chemical surge in our bodies. A controlled, calm response produces positive chemicals and results.

> "Exceptional patients
> have hope for
> the future and the
> perseverance to change
> in necessary ways."

We must participate fully in our own healing. Only when we develop a passionate involvement with all facets of life, including our illness, can we use all the tools at our disposal. Healing is a quest in self-discovery.

The Positive Patient

Be an Optimist

Few people would argue that pessimism is preferable to optimism. Most would not even be aware that optimists have better health. And even fewer yet would know how to change pessimistic behaviors into optimistic ones. Martin E. P. Seligman, Ph.D., author of *Learned Optimism: How to Change Your Mind and Your Life,* suggests that you can learn to be an optimist. He uses an ABC approach to look at our thought patterns. He shows that when humans encounter adversity, our thoughts solidify into beliefs, and those beliefs have consequences, and they dictate how we react to the original adversity. Once you become aware of that pattern, you can begin to change. The easiest approach is to keep notes of each problem or adversity in your life. Record them in a list. Then write down your beliefs at those moments. Finally, note the consequences, which are your feelings.

As an example, let's say you're trying to live a healthy lifestyle and lose some weight. You go to a friend's house for a meal and eat some things you shouldn't have. Afterward, you think that you blew it and go home and eat the last of the ice cream in the freezer. Your adversity is dealing with your weight, the challenge of a healthy lifestyle, and eating correctly. Because you consumed too much at the party, your belief is that your whole effort is ruined and that belief led you to eat the last of the ice cream, a consequence worse than your slight overindulgence at the party. (It's also a reminder to ban high-fat foods from your house. You might have to eat a yogurt next time.)

One method of altering your beliefs is to dispute them. Once you know you have a particular thought pattern and belief(s), you can work on this. In our previous example, the belief was that you blew it at the party. If you think about this logically, you will realize that you only overindulged a bit and certainly did not ruin a healthy lifestyle. If it happens again, you will consider your actions at the party a small detour on the road to wellness rather than a wreck.

Another method is to create a distraction from the adversity. Some people actually write the word "stop" on an index card and carry it with them all the time. If they are tempted by a cheeseburger, when they know they should have grilled chicken, they pull out the card and look at the word. If you simply try to get the cheeseburger out of your mind once it's there, you will hear nothing but "cheeseburger, cheeseburger, cheeseburger." You can also reinforce the word "stop" by slapping your hand on the table or wall and saying, "stop." You can use the word "no," or something else that's appropriate or distracting.

Staying Positive

Here are a few more simple suggestions to change negative situations into positive experiences.

See the silver linings—Always look for the good in a stressful or sad situation (reframing, in psychological terms). For instance, you just got fired. The positives might be that you hated your commute and can now work at home or closer to home, or you can now pursue your dream job, career, or educational opportunity. There is always a silver lining.

Enjoy small pleasures—Keep a journal of the good things that happen each day. Even on terrible days, and we all have them, something nice, good, or positive happens: the newspaper vendor liked your hat; the mango you had for a snack was at the peak of perfection; or the star-filled night sky was spectacular. On days when big pleasures come your way, mark the pages of your journal with sticky tabs or paper clips, or dog-ear the page. Then, on a bad day, go back and review the good days.

Redirect negative thoughts—You are stuck in line at the airport, a frequent occurrence for those who travel. Redirect your thinking from your pessimistic thoughts, such as "I'm never going to make my plane," to some pleasant memory. It could be your childhood memory of your grandmother baking bread or the more recent memory of walking in a fragrant garden. Make the choice to redirect negative thoughts to pleasant and positive ones.

Set reasonable goals—You can reinforce positive thinking by setting reasonable and achievable goals, then completing them. If you have trouble with this try limiting the number of things on your to-do list to ones that you can actually accomplish in a day. Break down large projects down into steps that you can complete. Instead of saying you will clean the garage today, make your goal to clean off the workbench. Doing this sets you up for success.

Be happy it's not worse—When things are going badly try to think of someone who has it worse. This is not about feeling superior; it's about deflecting negative thoughts. Everyone can probably remember a childhood moment when you complained to your mother about your shoes. She probably said something like, "Be happy; think of kids who don't have any shoes."

Fake it—Overcome down moments by simply faking it. Force yourself to smile and you will start to feel better—you know, "Turn that frown upside down." It's also true for laughing; just try to make yourself laugh and you will feel better.

Listen to happy music—Don't make your mood worse by listening to sad music. Find some "happy feet" music, any music that makes you smile, gets your foot tapping, or causes you to sing in the shower!

- Heart disease is a wake-up call to take care of our bodies. Nothing else has gotten us to eat better and exercise. Now we do!

- Heart disease causes patients, caregivers, family, and friends to realize how precious life is and how much we care about those we love and cherish. We show love and affection more.

- Heart disease motivates us to get up and do some of the things we have always wanted to try, to go to the places we have always wanted to see, to enjoy an adventure and realize some dreams. We understand how short life can be.

- Heart disease inspires us to count our blessings and to recognize the wonders of each new day.

- Heart disease motivates us to reach out to others who are dealing with the same disease and its side effects and share ways to cope and gain strength.

- Heart disease helps us find strength through new and existing support systems.

- Heart disease impels us to be concerned about the lifelong health of our children, grandchildren, other family, and friends.

- Heart disease causes us to learn to listen to our bodies.

- Heart disease inspires us to look to a higher power, to pray, and to meditate.

Follow Your Passion

"Hope deferred maketh the heart sick."
—PROVERBS 13:12

If you are unhappy with your job or career, you are unlikely to be happy over-all. Satisfaction with your job is critical to your health. Your illness is a reminder to follow your passions in life. We remember the poster from the 1960s that said, "Today is the first day of the rest of your life." Well, it really is. How many times have you heard about someone who kept his "nose to the grindstone" his whole life, amassing savings in order to "live it up" in retirement, only to die a few short months after getting his gold watch?

DARRELL'S STORY

"Each morning, I try to remind myself that I'm lucky—I'm still here, I'm alive—and to make the most of each day. I want to enjoy life and follow my passions, writing and gardening. I'm not sure where these will lead me, but I want to find out. I also want to remember to follow the advice of the country music song titled 'Live, Laugh, Love' each day."

"Nothing is so dear and precious as time."

—FRANÇOIS RABELAIS (C. 1490–1553), *Works*

HEART POINT

BE GOOD TO YOURSELF: Make a list of all the things that make you happy. Include everything from reading a book to cut flowers, scented candles, ripe mangoes, going to the movies or theater, going to the beach (with sunscreen), and so on. Every day, plan to do something from the list that makes you happy—live in the present. These small moments of happiness are evidence of taking control of your life. That is a major factor in life happiness and health.

It is important to live in the present and not worry about the future or past. Becoming the person you choose to be releases your creativity. You're able to go your own way and take risks in life.

ACCEPTING SPIRITUAL SUPPORT

IT WOULD BE very difficult to approach life without some sense of spirituality. A sense of spirituality moves us from looking only at our infinite beings to feeling a oneness with something and someone bigger than ourselves. It gives us the strength and serenity to keep going. Try to "keep a quiet place in your day." Find time every day to renew your spirit through prayer, meditation, nature, exercise, or experiences with people you love. A renewed spirit will better enable you to deal with the challenging times in life.

Spiritual Support

ELLEN'S STORY

"When I arrived at the hospital, my father was already in surgery. As I made my way to the waiting room, I was amazed at the crowd. There were too many people for everyone to cram into the room and find a place to sit down. They came to say they cared, and they came to say they were praying for my father and for our family. As a family with a heritage of faith, knowing that our 'family of faith' was praying calmed our fears and gave us hope and strength."

We know that the connection between body and spirit is age old, but more studies are being conducted to link faith and good health. In 1998, Duke University Medical Center doctors Harold Koenig and David Larson found that people who attended church on a regular basis every week were not as likely to end up in the hospital. If they were hospitalized, the study showed that they did not spend as much time there as those patients who went to church less or not at all. Some obvious reasons may be that regular church attendees tend to do less indulgent drinking, smoking, and risky sexual behavior. But just as important, an organized religious community tends to offer support and help to fellow parishioners. The study showed that people who are more isolated and have less support are more likely to do poorly physically and psychologically.

HEART POINT

A 1995 Dartmouth Medical School study found patients comforted by their faith had three times the chance of being alive six months after open-heart surgery than patients who found no comfort in religion.

We've devoted a lot of space in this book to helping you deal with stress because the medical world knows that stress impairs the immune system. Relying on prayer or meditation plus the support of friends can significantly reduce your stress level and foster a sense of peace. Remaining calm in the storm will give you a stronger sense of control and help you stay aware of your health needs.

The relaxation response, developed by Dr. Herbert Benson, uses a form of Transcendental Meditation™ that creates a specific physiological and mental state he calls relaxation. During the meditation, patients use abdominal breathing techniques, focus the mind in the present, and use a mantra, or specific focus for their elicitation. He found that more than 80 percent of the patients using the technique used a religious focus and many of the patients felt more spiritual after eliciting the relaxation response. The patients' efforts lowered their heart rate, blood pressure, metabolic rate, and breathing. He discovered that every major religion uses a type of simple and repetitive prayer. Benson concluded that those high in spirituality scored high in measures of psychological health, could raise their life-purpose index the most, and actually reduce pain.

Researchers in Italy have investigated rhythmic chanting and its effect on the heart. Repeating a yoga mantra or rosary prayer produces a calming effect on the heart. Before the chanting, the subject's respiratory rate was about fourteen breaths per minute. After reciting the yoga mantra or rosary, the subject's breathing rate dropped to about six breaths per minute, which has positive effects on respiratory and cardiovascular function.

Prayer

Most of the more than 88 percent of Americans who pray have a greater sense of well-being than those who don't. The majority has some sense of divine inspiration and has gone on to perform some specific action because of "God's instruction."

In a review of 212 health studies that looked at health and religious beliefs, noted by Dr. Robert Ivker and Edward Zorensky in *Thriving: The Complete*

Mind/Body Guide for Optimal Health and Fitness for Men, over 75 percent of the studies showed that individuals with religious commitments received health benefits from their beliefs. Regular prayer can reduce high blood pressure. Ivker and Zorensky suggested that prayer need not be formalized; you can simply tell your problems to God as you would a good friend. Or, pick a simple and well-known prayer, such as the Lord's Prayer, and repeat that a number of times.

Nature

Many great writers have described a spiritual connection to nature. Reread the words of Muir, Twain, Thoreau, and others as they describe the great natural wonders of the world. Garden writers transport us into colorful, fragrant, and peaceful vignettes in gardens or within a single flower. The painter Georgia O'Keefe connected powerfully and sensuously with nature with her flower paintings. Each of us has memories of our own special moments communing with nature.

DARRELL'S STORY

"Some of my memories of special moments in nature include: A night sky above Montauk Point Beach State Park so clear that a full moon seemed to light up the whole world, and billions and billions of stars twinkled above me as the Atlantic Ocean waves crashed ashore. A trickling brook flowed softly down Indian Head Mountain, a moss-covered hillside in the Catskill Mountains. A Hawaiian volcano blew red-hot sparks into the air and lava flowed into the deep blue sea. The silence of a quiet Iowa lake was broken by a fish jumping and splashing back into the water. Water tumbled and roared downward almost a mile from the top of Angel Fall into the tea-tinged Orinoco River below. A raptor soared and floated on warm air currents alongside the multicolored walls of Waimea Canyon on the island of Kauai, Hawaii."

Darrell's story here includes examples of the four elemental forms of nature: air, earth, fire, and water. Nature awakens and renews the senses. The more time you spend in nature the more ways you will find to connect with it spiritually. Start by spending as much time each day as you can outdoors. Walk through a park for exercise, garden, or sit quietly in a natural scenic spot or even in a man-made pocket park within the city. Watch the powerful movement of tides or the movement of a river. You can bathe in a mineral spring or slide into the warmth of a hot tub. Enjoy a campfire, build a fire in a fireplace, or even light a candle. Each of these actions helps you touch the spirit of nature.

BALANCING YOUR LIFE AND CAREGIVING

DOROTHY'S STORY
(caregiver, 75)

"I was raised in a poor family and had to work hard all my life. I have faced a lot of obstacles, so I thought that managing everything after my husband had heart surgery would be easy. I would not accept any help when he was in the hospital and only accepted food from friends when he came home. Those first weeks were hard. He didn't sleep much, which meant I didn't either. I had to do everything. What I discovered was that I made it through that beginning tough time, but after months and now a few years, I find myself needing someone to care about me. Maybe that sounds selfish, but it's how I feel. There is not a day that goes by that I don't think about my husband's condition and try to make sure he is eating right and we are exercising. I watch him all the time to be sure he is not overdoing things and getting stressed and tired. Many of my friends have already lost their husbands. I think about that every day too. Sometimes I just get tired of worrying and want someone to worry about me."

IN THIS STORY, we don't think Dorothy is selfish, we think she is honest and normal. We know that the way you relate to your patient depends largely on your environment, location, and relationship. But it doesn't matter if you are a cardiac patient's spouse, child, sibling, or friend, or whether you live nearby or long distance; you have two things in common:

♦ You must juggle the demands of your life while caring about someone you love who has heart disease.

♦ At some point in the caregiving journey, you are going to need support. The kind of support you need will differ. At times, you may need actual physical support to help you get things done so that you and your patient do not tackle too much. At other times, you will need emotional support. There are times when all of us need someone else to "prop us up" and let us use their shoulder for a while so that we can gain the strength to move forward.

There is no law that says you must do all the caregiving yourself plus handle anything else the patient can't handle during recovery or cannot do anymore. You will not get any award for taking on too much responsibility and too much worry. As we have stressed in other Star Points, it is crucial that you take care of yourself if you are going to be of any help to your patient. A 1997 survey from the National Family Caregivers Association found that two-thirds of caregivers experience some form of depression. So we say it again in this chapter, *get help!* Understand and accept that needing some assistance is normal.

This 1997 study reported the following information:

♦ 77 percent of caregivers have multiple responsibilities, including employment, childcare, and household maintenance.

♦ 65 percent of family caregivers do not receive consistent help from family members.

♦ 69 percent of caregivers say frustration is their most frequently felt emotion.

♦ 49 percent of all caregivers say they have suffered from prolonged depression.

♦ Over 40 percent of caregivers consider the loss of leisure time, feelings of isolation, and the change in family dynamics to be the most burdensome aspects of caregiving.

♦ 30 percent of caregivers feel taken for granted by their loved ones, while 46 percent feel appreciated.

♦ Over 80 percent of caregivers are women.

♦ 54 percent care for a spouse or partner.

♦ 21 percent care for a parent.

♦ 17 percent care for a child.

Even choosing to be positive and renewing your spirit daily can become overwhelming for a caregiver. Caregiving is not easy. It is an act of love that requires constant reevaluation. No matter how much you want to help and care for someone you love, you must balance the other demands of your life with your caregiving. If your caregiving role remained constant and the same each day, then it would be easier to balance with the rest of your life. But when you are the caregiver for a heart disease patient, your role will change as your patient's health changes. You move from being caretaker back to caregiver. You may go through long periods of time when your main caregiving role consists of checking in with your patient about blood pressure or diet. There will be periods of time for many caregivers when only a doctor's appointment acts as a reminder that they live with or care for a heart disease patient. But the common denominators for caregivers of heart disease patients is their constant concern for their patient's well-being and the challenge of balancing their own lives.

Emergency Caregiving

In many cases, discovering your friend or loved one has heart disease begins with the news of his heart attack or her immediate need for bypass surgery. There is not much time to get your "ducks in a row." Think through what you need to take care of in order to drop everything and care for a post-op patient. Dealing with heart disease lasts a lifetime. Your first time to deal with a heart emergency may not be your last. Be prepared.

At home:

- Who do you need to call and enlist to help with your family?
- Can someone else manage the children?
- What events are coming up in the next week or two that you need to make preparations for in your absence?
- If your caregiving requires you to leave town, tell a trusted friend and a neighbor that you will be gone. Give them numbers where you can be reached. Call someone to pick up your newspaper and mail.
- Talk to your children about your friend or relative's condition. Explain why you are needed to help. Enlist your children's and spouse's support to help out at home. They may feel more a part of your caregiving if you encourage them to make cards for the patient or to pray for him or her.
- Assure family at home that you will call regularly to let them know the patient's condition and to check on how they are doing.

At work:

- Who do you need to notify about your situation and to check on how much time off you can take?
- Ask if you can take time off with pay or if your company makes special allowances when you must take time off for the illness of a family member.
- Think through dates and deadlines for the next two weeks. Line up coworkers who can substitute for you or keep things going until you return.
- Can you check your phone messages when you are away or do you need to change your voice mail to alert callers that you are gone?
- Leave numbers where you can be reached.
- Take a laptop computer so you can work or check your e-mail while away.
- Set times when you will call in and check on things at the office.

Ongoing Caregiving

Caregivers can face many problems dealing with their patients, their kids, careers, spouses, and their own health. After you face the post-op crisis, what do you need to consider as your caregiving role continues?

- Be ready to move from caretaker to caregiver. Let go of doing everything for the patient. Allow him or her to resume normal activities following doctor's orders. Allow others to move into the role as caregiver.
- Do you need to line up home health care for your patient if you have to resume working? Remind yourself that it's okay if you need to get professional assistance or enlist the help of other family members and friends. You cannot do it all.
- Will the situation require the patient to move in with you? If you are married or have children, make the decisions and family adjustments together. Make everyone a part of the caregiving team. Understand that change is never easy for anyone of any age. Be sensitive to your spouse's and children's feelings, but remember that you must take care of yourself or you will be of no use to care for anyone else. Ongoing communication about how you feel and how other family members feel is crucial to you and your patient's well-being. Hold regular family meetings to talk about teamwork and changes.
- If you continue to work, what kinds of options do you have? If you need to take more time off to stay at home with a patient or to accompany a patient to medical appointments, what arrangements can you make. Talk to your employer about different options. Can you move to a flex-time schedule? Can you work from home more? Does the Family and Medical Leave Act apply to you? Ask your employer. The Act entitles eligible employees to a maximum of twelve weeks a year of unpaid leave for family caregiving without loss of job security or health benefits. Due to a variety of restrictions, carefully check what you are eligible for through your company.
- As we have stressed throughout this book, take regularly scheduled time out for yourself. Take care of your own emotional, physical, mental, and

spiritual health. It is as much at risk as the patient's health. Eat right, exercise, rest, reduce stress, and renew your spirit.

Long-Distance Caregiving

You may not be the main caregiver, but if you have a loved one with heart disease, you can provide support. How can you help in providing care for a loved one who does not live in the same city?

- ◆ Keep up with the doctor appointments and medications. After each doctor's visit, ask the patient to give you a report.
- ◆ Keep a journal or log of the patient's health. This will help you see any patterns that are caused by medications or activities.
- ◆ Insist on helping. Some patients or main caregivers may not want to inconvenience other family members or friends, but they will need your help and support all along the journey.
- ◆ Call frequently and check on the main caregiver. Allow him or her to share feelings and vent. When possible, schedule a visit and offer to relieve the caregiver with some respite time.
- ◆ If you feel that the patient and main caregiver are not asking doctors enough questions or the right questions, call the doctor. It would not be good for several family members to do the same thing, but one appointed person can call to make sure the patient is getting the best care. Have a list of questions ready to ask the doctor or nurse when you call.
- ◆ Talk to the patient and listen to his or her feelings. Even though it may seem that roles have been reversed, the patient is an adult who must learn how to live a healthy life with a lifelong disease. As long as the patient is mentally competent, allow the patient to make his or her own decisions. However, your encouragement accompanied by your efforts at living a healthier lifestyle will have a positive influence on the patient.

Recognize that you need support too. It is stressful to deal with someone's care long distance. Develop your own support system of friends, other relatives, medical personnel you can direct your questions to, and other people who are long-distance caregivers.

ELLEN'S STORY

"Being a long-distance secondary caregiver can be frustrating. It is that frustration that motivated me to coauthor this book. I have found that finding other caregivers to talk with makes such a difference. And perhaps the best help has come in talking with Darrell and other people who live with heart disease every day. I have found patients and caregivers at the office, at church, in the mall, on airplanes, at the doctor's office, and just about everywhere I go. Hearing the stories of both sides has helped me understand how important the caregiver–patient partnership is and how important it is for both to find ongoing support."

Take advantage of the great information organizations and agencies offer. In Resources we list numerous organizations and websites. In addition, many hospitals offer ongoing seminars and support groups for caregivers.

AFFECT THE HEALTH OF FAMILY *and* FRIENDS

WOMEN AND HEART DISEASE

A WARNING TO WOMEN

HEART DISEASE HAS always been considered a man's disease. In a recent survey by the American Heart Association only 8 percent of women considered it their major health threat. The same survey showed that 74 percent of women between the ages of twenty-five and thirty-four believe that cancer is their biggest threat to good health. Even more shocking, in a 1995 Gallup Survey, more than one in three primary care doctors did not know that heart disease is the major killer of women. The real facts follow:

- Heart disease is the number-one killer of women.
- Heart disease causes 44.4 percent of all female deaths in the United States.
- More than 2 million women have had a stroke.
- Over 93,000 women die of stroke each year.
- One in ten American women has some form of heart disease.
- One in four women over sixty-five has heart disease.
- Over 9 million women suffer from some form of heart disease.
- Over 234,000 females die from heart disease each year, 43,000 from breast cancer, and 61,700 from lung cancer.

These facts, compiled from National Institutes of Health and American Heart Association statistics, are shocking to most people. When you consider that all of the female deaths annually from accidents, AIDS, diabetes, pneumonia, chronic lung disease, and all forms of cancer still total fewer than the deaths from coronary heart disease, you begin to understand the magnitude of the problem.

TREATMENT OF WOMEN

A FRIEND'S MOTHER is a slim, vibrant fifty-four year old who exercised and ate a healthy diet. When she went to her doctor complaining of chest pains, he treated her for indigestion and sent her home. Two days later she was taken to the hospital by ambulance with a substantial heart attack and is now fighting hard to regain her life. Unfortunately, this is a rather typical story of women and heart disease. Heart disease is the major killer of women, yet is not taken seriously by many doctors. A number of studies have documented some serious differences in health care provided to men and women with heart complications. Heart disease is generally diagnosed at a later stage in women than in men, is more serious, and is treated less aggressively. Even when the medical tests show significant signs of heart disease, fewer women than men are referred for bypass surgery. The American Heart Association says that of women who have heart attacks, 42 percent die within one year compared to 24 percent of the men.

WOMEN'S SYMPTOMS

ONE PROBLEM OF diagnosing women with heart disease is atypical symptoms, symptoms that are often very different from male symptoms. One woman went to bed around midnight and started feeling an uncomfortable and peculiar prickly sensation. After two nights of the odd feeling, she went to her doctor. She learned later that she had had a heart attack.

Another woman, Nancy Loving, at age forty-eight, woke up one night with a cold, clammy feeling, light-headedness, and upper back pain. She thought she had the flu. It simply did not occur to her that she was having a heart attack, in spite of a family history of heart disease, smoking, and being overweight. She was lucky. She just felt that something was terribly wrong (another symptom for women) and went to the emergency room. She was fortunate to have a doctor who recognized her symptoms of heart attack. She avoided major heart damage because of the accurate diagnosis and action by the doctor.

Nancy cofounded the women's support group Womenheart with two other women who were not as lucky. When Jackie Markham had symptoms, her diagnosis was flu, and she was told to go back home and rest. The next day she had a major heart attack, which was misdiagnosed again. Finally a female doctor reviewed her chart and realized that she had had a heart attack, but by then, 10 percent of her heart muscle had died. Ambulance drivers refused to transport Judy Mingram to the hospital, mistakenly thinking she had a cocaine overdose. At forty years old, she ended up having an emergency bypass.

Though some women have symptoms most people associate with heart attacks—substantial or crushing chest pain—they are more likely to have less typical symptoms. Not all men have typical symptoms either, though

HEART POINT

After Nancy Loving's heart attack, she sought support from other women with heart disease. Finding none, she cofounded, with Jackie Markham and Judy Mingram, Womenheart (www.women-heart.com), an organization dedicated to educating and supporting women with heart disease.

heart disease is still a more likely diagnosis for them. There certainly is a problem with diagnosing heart disease in women. A major component of the problem must be the mistaken impression that women are at lower risk for heart disease. Younger women do have some protection from hormones, but as women age, their risk levels quickly catch up to those of men. More than one in seven women aged forty-five to sixty-four show some sign of heart disease. After age sixty-five, a woman's risk equals a man's risk of heart disease; one in four dies from it.

A significant problem for women is having the possibility of heart disease taken seriously. You need to have an excellent understanding of your own body. You need to listen to your body and respond appropriately. Women often have less specific symptoms or ones that can mimic other common diseases such as the flu. Some possible symptoms include:

♦ Pressure, squeezing, tightness, fullness, or discomfort in the center of the chest that may, or may not, radiate to arms, neck, or back. This may be intermittent or linger for several minutes. If the pain or pressure continues for over fifteen minutes, call 911.

♦ Pain or pressure in arms, neck, shoulders, or upper back, no chest involvement. If a man has back pain, he will normally get an EKG and X-ray. As women age, the risk of heart problems and the need for similar treatment is increased.

♦ Dizziness, light-headedness, fainting, or blackouts. (There is a major difference in how people perceive someone fainting, depending on gender. With a man, people are likely to wonder, "Heart attack?"; for a woman, people are likely to get her a glass of water.)

♦ Irregular heartbeats, abnormal heart rhythm, palpitations, or skipping beats.

♦ Shortness of breath or difficulty breathing. Don't ignore ongoing shortness of breath when you are vacuuming, climbing stairs, etc. Smoking will make it worse.

♦ Unexplained fatigue or exhaustion. A patient typically has diminishing energy over a period of a few weeks, maybe thinking she has the flu; then she experiences some type of chest pain.

♦ Paleness, clammy sweats, or excessive sweating. Women are less likely to describe sweating as a problem; they seem embarrassed by the symptom. Consider describing it as a substantial increase in perspiration; certainly describe it to your doctor.

♦ Nausea or intense indigestion (no relief with antacids).

♦ Feelings of impending doom.

♦ Abdominal bloating. Many women experience bloating during their menstrual cycle but it also can be a warning for heart disease. Be vigilant for bloating during or immediately after vigorous activity of any kind.

♦ A change in ability to think, or becoming confused (particularly true for African American women).

♦ Suddenly developing vision difficulties.

♦ Discomfort when lying down.

CHRISTINE'S STORY
(heart patient, 54)

"I was active and energetic, working out or walking most days. I danced and swam frequently. One day I felt terrible, my stomach hurt, I was nauseous, felt weak, and clammy, and was short of breath. I went to my doctor, who gave me an EKG that didn't show anything. He sent me home with an antacid and a diagnosis of 'upset stomach.' Three days later, I was in the hospital with a substantial heart attack. Let this be a warning to all women: 'Follow your feelings.' I knew something was wrong but didn't push hard enough. I don't want that to happen to any other woman."

Speed of treatment is critical for anyone, woman or man, having a heart attack. Get to know your body (Star Point One describes how to do that), then trust your instincts, then insist on the possibility of heart attack. You may not be correct, but can you afford to be wrong? Often, a woman's first confirmed symptom of heart disease is death. If you end up in the emergency room or at a doctor's office with any of the previously mentioned symptoms, insist that medical personnel consider a heart attack as a possibility.

> "Often, a woman's first confirmed symptom of heart disease is death."

SUE'S STORY
(heart patient, 66)

"I have coronary artery disease that required bypass surgery. I also have unstable angina. I had almost no symptoms, but my primary doctor recognized the problem before I had a heart attack. My initial reaction was, 'Not me! I am a woman and this is a man's disease and I am only fifty-six years old.' The only risk factor I had was stress. It has been hard for me to adjust to life with heart disease. After ten years, I am still learning how to live with it."

WOMEN AND HEART DISEASE STUDIES

UNTIL RECENTLY, MOST studies of heart disease have been conducted with men. For every twenty-five men who participated in a heart disease study, only one woman did the same. Women were excluded because of hormonal differences and monthly fluctuations. In another sad truth, perhaps researchers also believed the lie that heart disease was a man's disease. Consequently, study results may not apply to women. Many new studies will include women, and the results will be extremely helpful.

RISK FACTORS

WE DISCUSSED RISK factors in previous chapters. In the following section we outline those factors again and deal with the significant differences between men and women.

There are some parallels in risk factors between men and women. It's true for both that the risk of heart disease increases quickly when you have multiple risk factors. You have no control over some risk factors such as age and family history. You can control or lessen the impact of others, such as obesity, smoking, sedentary lifestyle, high blood pressure, high LDL cholesterol, and diabetes, as men can. Because women live longer than men do, it's crucial to do all you can to modify your life to minimize these risks. The results of the Harvard Nurses' Health Study (described later in this section) provide another incentive—for about two-thirds of those women who died suddenly from a heart attack, it was their first symptom. If you have several of the following risk factors it should be a "wake-up call" to improve your lifestyle and your chances.

Age

As women age, their risk of heart disease increases. Women seem to lag behind men by about ten to fifteen years. By the age of forty-five, risk starts to increase until age sixty-five, when the risk equals a man's. African American women's risk of heart disease is worse than for Caucasian women. At age twenty-five, heart disease is the number-one killer of African American women.

HEART POINT

At age 65, female and male risk of heart disease is equal.

As we age, our bodies are less able to handle certain challenges. Cholesterol levels increase with age. Glucose intolerance can become adult onset diabetes. A woman's body produces less estrogen after menopause. Many believe that hormones provide a certain protection from heart disease.

Heart disease does not just appear overnight; it builds slowly over many years. Artery-clogging plaque starts to accumulate early in life. Autopsies were used to study a group of young women, age fifteen to thirty-four, who died from accidents, suicide, or murder. Their arteries already were accumulating plaque, which eventually leads to heart disease. Lifestyle choices have a great impact on your health.

Family History

Family history of heart disease is an equally important risk factor for women and men. The importance for women may come from the early warning it provides. Women live longer and develop heart disease later in life than men. The early warning of a family history of heart disease gives women more years to act, improve their lifestyle, and reverse the onset of disease.

The magnitude of risk is determined by how closely related the relatives are and how early they experienced disease or had a heart attack. The greatest risk is when your brother or father had a heart attack before the age of fifty-five or your sister or mother before the age of sixty.

The danger extends to risk factors for heart disease: diabetes, hypertension, high LDL cholesterol, and obesity. If any close relatives suffer with any of those conditions, you need to inform your doctors, be diligent in monitoring your health, and begin lifestyle modifications to improve your odds of not developing those problems.

Obesity

Obesity is a risk factor that adds to other problems. It makes your LDL cholesterol higher and your HDL lower. Blood pressure drops if you lose weight. Blood sugar also diminishes with a decrease in weight. As detailed in Star Point Five, there is an epidemic of obesity in America today, with more than half the population overweight or obese.

The Harvard Nurses' Health Study looked at the lifestyles of more than 120,000 women. This comprehensive study began in 1976 and continues to monitor the impact of lifestyle choices on these women. The results indicate that women who gained even small amounts of weight after their teen years increased their risk of a heart attack. The greater the weight gain, the greater the risk.

Body Mass Index (BMI) is one of the best measures of determining your body fat. (Instructions can be found in Star Point Five.) As BMI increases so does your risk of adult onset diabetes along with increasing blood pressure. A BMI in the overweight range (25 – < 30) also increases the risk of breast cancer in postmenopausal women, pulmonary embolism, endometrial cancer, gallstones, kidney stones, and arthritis. The Nurses' Health Study also suggests the possible increase in risk for ovarian cancer, asthma, and cataracts.

HEART POINT

Women who are apple-shaped have greater risk of cancer, diabetes, hypertension, and stroke than those who are pear-shaped.

A high BMI also affects your quality of life. It stands to reason, and is backed up by study results, that being obese or overweight hinders a woman's ability to function. The more overweight someone is, the more difficult it is to handle day-to-day tasks normally.

The study also shows that obese women (BMI 30 and greater) are four times more likely to die of cardiovascular disease than women with a healthy BMI (25 is healthy).

Physical Inactivity

Physical inactivity is a separate risk factor that also affects several other risk factors. The more active you are, the less likely you are to be overweight. Exercise also benefits blood glucose, blood pressure, and cholesterol. The Surgeon General recommends thirty minutes of moderate exercise on most days of the week. Even three ten-minute segments are beneficial. Find some activity you enjoy doing and it will seem so much easier. Examples of moderate activity include gardening, walking, bicycling, raking leaves, or yard work.

HEART POINT

Female smokers with angina often respond inadequately to angina medications and don't do as well after bypass surgery as nonsmokers.

Smoking

Smoking is a major killer of men and women. We describe the problems and some suggestions for stopping in Star Point Five. Unfortunately, more women have begun to smoke in recent years. There are now more young females than males smoking. This will have great consequence in years ahead.

High Blood Pressure

Even slight elevations in blood pressure increase risk of heart disease for women. In general, a woman's blood pressure runs much lower than a man's until age fifty-five. After that, women and men tend to have similar levels. The chance of high blood pressure is much greater after the age of forty-five, and by age fifty-five, more women than men have high blood pressure.

Optimal readings are <120/<80, normal is <130/<85, and high normal is 130–139/85–89. Several readings should be taken as blood pressure varies by time of day, mood, and stress level. Some people have "white-coat hypertension," an elevated blood pressure while in the doctor's office.

BLOOD PRESSURE LEVEL IN MM HG

CATEGORY	SYSTOLIC	DIOSTOLIC
Optimal	<120	<80
Normal	<130	<85
High-normal	130–139	85–89
Hypertension		
Stage 1	140–159	90–99
Stage 2	160–179	100–109
Stage 3	≥180	≥110

Source: The Sixth Report of the Joint National committee on Detection,Evaluation, and Treatment of High Blood Pressure, NIH, NHLBI, 1997

High normal and higher blood pressure readings require action. Many studies have established the link between high blood pressure and coronary heart disease. The Nurses' Health Study found that women with high blood pressure had 3.5 times the risk of coronary heart disease and six times the risk of a fatal heart attack compared to women with normal blood pressure.

The first step to fighting high blood pressure is making lifestyle improvements. At levels above 160/100 doctors will probably recommend medications along with lifestyle changes. Lose weight if necessary to reach a healthy weight level and maintain that level. Eat a diet high in fruits, vegetables, and whole grains and low in fat. Limit your salt intake. Some individuals are more salt sensitive than others are. Stop smoking and become physically active.

HEART POINT

Cholesterol

High total cholesterol, high LDL ("bad") cholesterol, and low HDL ("good") cholesterol are risk factors for heart disease for women and men. Desirable levels for the general population are total cholesterol under 200 mg/dl and LDL cholesterol under 130 mg/dl. If you have heart disease, had a heart attack, or have two other risk factors for heart disease, the

Total Lipid Profile: Women should ask for a total lipid profile in order to know their specific readings of LDL and HDL cholesterol and triglycerides. Knowing total cholesterol is not enough.

recommended target level is LDL cholesterol of 100 mg/dl or less. Lifestyle factors—weight, diet, smoking, and physical activity levels—affect cholesterol.

HDL cholesterol works to "clean out" your arteries; consequently, more is better. Levels of 60 mg/dl are protective against heart disease, while readings of 35 mg/dl and less are a major risk factor for heart disease. Low HDL levels are more detrimental for women, doubling the relative risk (men's risk level increases by 46 percent). HDL levels are more difficult to change than LDL levels. (Read all the recommendations in Star Point Five). Each increase of 1 mg/dl is likely to produce a 3.2 percent decrease in risk.

High blood triglyceride levels, over 250 mg, are also more of a problem for women and more likely to predict heart disease. Improved lifestyle also helps lower them.

Diabetes

Diabetes is bad for men, even worse for women. Diabetic women are likely to have high blood pressure, high cholesterol, and to be overweight. They

HEART POINT

Over 70 percent of diabetics die from some form of cardiovascular disease or heart problems.

HEART POINT

If you are overweight, have a family history of diabetes, over age forty-four, African American, Asian, Hispanic, or Native American, developed gestational diabetes during a pregnancy, gave birth to a baby weighing over nine pounds, have high blood pressure (140/90 or higher), HDL cholesterol of 35 mg/dl or lower, or triglyceride level of 250 mg/dl or higher, have your glucose levels checked at least once per year. Get tested if you have any of these warning signs: frequent urination, increased thirst, and fatigue.

are two times as likely to suffer a heart attack. They often also have dulled pain sensations and may not feel a heart attack.

Birth Control Pills

The high-dose estrogen birth control pills of the past used to increase the risk of heart disease, especially for women who smoked. Today, most birth control pills use a low dose of estrogen, 35 micrograms or less. At that level there is minimal risk for most women. If you are a smoker, however, it would be best to consider another form of birth control. Birth control pills may increase blood pressure. If you have high blood pressure or develop it, discuss alternatives with your doctor. Anyone who already has some form of heart disease or cardiovascular disease should inform her doctor before he or she prescribes birth control pills.

Stress and Emotional Issues

We know, as discussed in other sections of this book, that stress can have a significant negative impact on men. Again, most of the specific stress research and observational studies with coronary-prone personalities and life stresses were done with men, though results suggest a similar result.

New research reported by Jay Kaplan,

Ph.D., Wake Forest University Baptist Medical Center, suggests that women who have reduced estrogen levels in premenopausal years are at higher risk for heart disease. Animal studies, with female monkeys, indicate that stress levels affect estrogen levels. These studies suggest that premenopausal women with high stress levels are at a substantial risk of heart disease. This could begin to explain a continuing study of autopsy results. More than one-third of women, by the age of thirty-five, have significant atherosclerosis in their coronary arteries. This evidence is a warning to women to control stress throughout their lives.

We cannot avoid all stress in life; the secret is to minimize or manage it. A few bad days or individual events will not produce terrible consequences. Ongoing and unrelenting stress will ravage your body. As women's role in society continues to change they must be vigilant in managing their stress. Greater numbers of women in the workplace are juggling families, caring for children and parents at the same time, and managing households. The number of divorces continues to be high, producing many single moms facing these challenges. This runs counter to research that suggests that supportive relationships lower the chance of developing heart disease and prolong life following a heart attack.

Sex is not only a part of loving and supportive relationships but also appears to contribute to maintaining a healthy heart. Dr. Alexander Lowen, author of *Love, Sex, and Your Heart,* suggests that, for women, an unsatisfying sex life is a risk factor for heart disease.

Anger and hostility are problems for women as well as men. Unexpressed anger may be worse yet. Evidence continues to mount that it leads women to develop and die from heart disease.

Women experiencing extreme worry and anxiety have a high risk of heart disease. Add hostility to the mix and the women are more than 40 percent more likely to develop heart disease than women without hostility.

Many women now find themselves in the role of caregiver. Being part of the "sandwich" generation, they may have an ill spouse, ailing parents, and children in college. Preliminary results from the Nurses' Health Study suggest that a woman spending nine or more hours a week caring for an ill spouse may have an 80 percent greater risk of heart disease than someone not in that role. Women caring for grandchildren nine or more hours per week had a surprising 55 percent increase in risk.

In some ways women are better able to handle stress. They seem much more willing to communicate frustrations to friends. They are also able to cry more freely. Women also seem much more likely to try yoga, meditation, and other stress reduction techniques than men are. Efforts to release stress and control anger are likely to pay off in the future.

Depression

Depression may be a separate risk factor for women. Some doctors think that depression is a severe form of stress. Levels of the hormones norepinephrine and cortisol, which push blood pressure and heart rate higher than normal, are elevated in depressed individuals. Over time depression causes arteries to narrow. According to a Danish study, women who are depressed are as much as 70 percent more likely to have a heart attack, compared to women who aren't.

We are not talking about a few bad days or short-term sadness; they can be overcome with meditation, exercise, or other relaxation techniques. Check the following list to see if symptoms apply to you or a friend or loved one. Consider seeking out professional help if three or more apply.

ONGOING SIGNS OF DEPRESSION

♦ Overeating, overdrinking alcohol, or loss of appetite
♦ Sleep patterns disrupted: too little or too much sleep
♦ Feeling empty, guilty, or worthless
♦ Feeling sad or hopeless
♦ Difficulty making decisions or concentrating
♦ Apathy or fatigue
♦ Irritability

TESTING FOR HEART DISEASE

THE EXERCISE STRESS test, or treadmill stress test, is a problem for women. The test results in many false indications of heart disease. Some experts suggest that as many as 40 percent of the tests are inaccurate. The test was created and perfected for men; that may explain part of the problem. The high-speed scans to measure calcium in arteries are also less reliable for women. Women's arteries do not calcify at the same rate men's do. Higher-accuracy tests for women include a stress echo (exercise echocardiogram) and the thallium stress test.

IMPROVE YOUR LIFESTYLE, EXTEND YOUR LIFE

IMPROVING YOUR LIFESTYLE can produce astounding benefits. The Nurses' Health Study predicts that you can reduce your risk of heart disease by 82 percent with the following improvements:

♦ Don't smoke and avoid secondhand smoke.
♦ Avoid becoming overweight.
♦ Exercise thirty minutes seven days per week (any vigorous exercise equivalent to brisk walking; exercise can be unevenly spaced in ten-minute intervals).
♦ Drink alcohol moderately (no more than two drinks per day).
♦ Eat a healthy diet, including at least five servings of fruit and vegetables each day; include whole grains/high-fiber foods, plenty of folate, and fish.
♦ Take a daily, low-dose aspirin.

HORMONE REPLACEMENT THERAPY

THE RECOMMENDATION UNTIL recently has been for postmenopausal women to use hormone replacement therapy (HRT) to help prevent heart attacks and disease. The prevailing wisdom was that a woman's natural hormones provided the protecting mechanism against heart problems until menopause, and HRT would do the same after. Research now shows that HRT does not seem to protect women against heart disease. The American Heart Association now suggests that healthy women not take hormones after menopause to prevent heart disease and those with heart disease should not start them.

HRT therapy may still be valuable for other reasons, such as symptomatic relief from menopausal problems, or to combat other health issues. Follow the research in these areas, discuss the issue with your doctor, and decide the best course for you.

TAKE CHARGE OF YOUR LIFE

WE ENCOURAGE WOMEN to become exceptional patients and take charge of their health and heart care. Many doctors still don't consider heart disease a major problem for women. If your doctor feels that way, change doctors. You need to be able to communicate and be an equal partner in your entire health care, including your heart. If you ever have to go to the emergency room with symptoms that might be a heart attack, tell medical personnel of the possibility and insist on appropriate treatment.

ELLEN'S STORY

"I have experienced the caregiver role, along with my mother, who lives with my father, a heart disease patient. But I had a scare while writing this book that allowed me to see what it is like from a patient's point of view. It was Thanksgiving and we were writing the section dealing with the signs and symptoms of heart disease. I read where women were more hesitant to go to the emergency room or the doctor with their symptoms because they didn't want to appear foolish or look like they were 'crying wolf.'

"On Thanksgiving Day, I started developing some strange symptoms. I felt awful. I didn't really want to eat what I had spent the morning cooking, which is unusual for me. That evening I felt even worse. I started having a pain in my chest area, and over the next day it moved down my arm and neck and back. I felt nauseated and like I had been run over by an eighteen-wheeler. I tried antacids and pain relievers and got no real relief. After almost three days of this and very little sleep, my daughter convinced me to go to the emergency room. I had actually considered driving myself and not waking her up. (As I relayed that to Darrell, he reminded me, in his always subtle way, how stupid and dangerous that could have been. We all need honest friends to say what we need to hear!)

"I took the time to write down my symptoms on a piece of paper so I could communicate clearly at the hospital. You have to understand that I hate to go to hospitals and doctors. I have a high vegal nerve response that causes me to pass out, have a seizure, and have my heart rate and blood pressure drop incredibly low when I am stuck with needles. So, I was not excited to go at all. Fortunately, the ER staff was extremely helpful and quick. We barely sat five minutes in the waiting room before they took me back.

"After blood work, an EKG, and a chest X-ray, the attending ER physician concluded that it was not a heart attack and referred me to my primary doctor. He was very helpful—discussing symptoms and possible other causes with me and stressing that sometimes a woman's heart problems are not caught by the usual methods.

"As I sat on the bed all hooked up to monitors, I just kept thinking how much I didn't want to know about the patient side of heart disease. I liked being a caregiver and wanted to stay that way!

"What did I learn? I learned that even when I knew all about what to do, as a woman, I was hesitant to believe that I should really go and see what was going on with me. I learned that a hospital would take me seriously and that being able to describe my symptoms helped. I took an aspirin at home, knowing that it would help to counter a heart attack if I was having one. I learned that giving an aspirin is standard procedure in the ER if there is any suspicion someone is having a heart attack. I learned that when I am faced with an emergency situation, I'd better have a plan and follow through with it. Even though I was not having a heart attack, I modeled for my daughter what anyone should do if they are experiencing symptoms. I hope she learned from the experience that heart disease is real. It could affect her mom and it could affect her.

"And yes—for your information, I did pass out in the ER!"

TEACH YOUR CHILDREN WELL

"My mother died of cancer and my dad is battling congestive heart failure. I don't want their lives or their suffering to be in vain. I am taking better care of myself. My dad's health problems are a result of the way he lived when he was my age. I've started talking with my teenage boys about a healthy lifestyle. They have their whole lives ahead of them. If they live right starting now, it will be a long, healthier life."

> "The genetic tentacles of risk reach all the offspring and siblings of anyone with some form of heart disease."

A STANDARD RISK factor for heart problems is a family history of cardiovascular disease. With over 50 million people with heart disease, the statistics of family members who are at risk are staggering. The genetic tentacles of risk reach all the offspring and siblings of anyone with some form of heart disease. Conservatively, that means that over 75 million additional Americans are at increased risk for heart disease. With the increasing prevalence of obesity, high-fat diets, diabetes, and a sedentary lifestyle, the risk of heart disease may reach 75 percent of the adult population. Those with elevated blood pressure, LDL cholesterol, and homocysteine levels are likely to pass those risks on to their offspring. Parents are also likely to teach, by example, bad habits that lead to heart disease: inactive lifestyle, bad eating habits, and high-stress behaviors.

Dr. William Franklin, clinical assistant professor of medicine at Georgetown University Medical School, suggests that those with a family history of heart disease should be aggressively treated to prevent heart attacks. He thinks testing should be begun at an early age and that we should focus on prevention for those at risk. There is recent evidence that the problem continues to worsen, and the huge amount of heart disease in older Americans is now affecting younger Americans. A new study showed that more than 3 percent of fifteen- to nineteen-year-old males have significant blockages from cholesterol plaque in their arteries, the results from autopsies of individuals killed in auto and other accidents. The percentages increase in slightly older men, with 19 percent of those in the thirty- to thirty-four age group showing plaque. Plaque can cause atherosclerosis, heart attacks, and strokes. Some authorities suggest these blockage levels should be treated with cholesterol-lowering drugs. It would be so much better to avoid the problem and teach children to live a heart-smart lifestyle.

HEART POINT

More than 22 percent of teenagers between the ages of twelve and seventeen are overweight.

In January 2000, U.S. Surgeon General David Satcher bemoaned the decrease in physical education in schools. He suggested that this accounts for the epidemic of childhood obesity that will lead to increased illness, disability, and premature death. There is a link between childhood and adult obesity. Obesity leads to increased risk of diabetes and heart disease. He created a ten-year initiative called "Healthy People 2010." The plan aims to reduce obesity in children and to double the number of children who exercise at least thirty minutes per day. Preventing adult heart attacks begins in childhood.

Parents should focus on teaching children how to eat a healthy and balanced diet, not on weight. Early adolescence is a critical and challenging time. Children are developing their sense of self-worth. Making weight the issue, instead of healthy living, could create a body image problem and lower their self-esteem.

TELL YOUR STORY OFTEN

ELLEN'S STORY

"When I finally caught on that I was at risk of heart disease, I started preaching about it to my own two children and to my nieces. It's hard to take the image of a grandfather in ICU and translate that to your own life, which still seems invincible. I want them to know that it's up to them to break the cycle of heart disease in our family just like it is up to me. They can choose to eat healthy and live healthy. They can choose how they deal with stress and set lifelong good habits. Although it has not been easy for my parents to deal with my father's heart disease and complications, their struggles remain as a constant reminder to the rest of the family that we MUST take care of ourselves beginning NOW."

HEART POINT

The average teenager drinks 65 gallons of soft drinks per year, which includes approximately 3,000 teaspoons of sugar and 48,000 calories, adding to the epidemic of obesity and Type 2 diabetes.

THE MORE YOU discuss your heart problems with friends and family the more impact you will have. Everyone will listen when you are going through surgery. That always gets their attention. After the surgery their interest level is likely to diminish, but keep at it; you never know when you will get through to someone.

Write Down Your Story

It's a good idea to record your story. It will become interesting family history along with a record of your exact medical conditions. A family medical history is very useful for future generations. Many diseases and conditions have a genetic component. This will help your grandchildren and their children.

ENCOURAGE PROPER MEDICAL EVALUATIONS

MANY INDIVIDUALS AVOID doctors and regular examinations. This is bad enough when everyone is healthy, but becomes dangerous when there are patterns of risk within families. Many risk factors for heart disease can be passed from generation to generation. High blood pressure, cholesterol, and triglyceride levels are particularly critical for children and siblings of individuals with those conditions.

CHANGE FAMILY TRADITIONS

UNHEALTHY FAMILY TRADITIONS should be changed. We are not suggesting that you need to do away with everything your mother or grandmother (or father) prepared for special occasions and holidays. There are many ways to change holiday dinners into healthy meals.

Avoid Using Food as a Reward

Do not give food to your children as a reward for achievement or good behavior. Find other ways to reinforce success and accomplishment. Try small gifts such as books, CDs, or tickets to a movie.

Educate by Example

Living a healthy lifestyle is the single most powerful thing you can do to improve others' lives in addition to your own. People are often surprised and amazed at what you do to improve your health. They say to Darrell, "You eat no meat?" or "You walk how many miles each day?" They learn how you deal with the threat of heart disease. They are far more likely to follow your example rather than respond to some statistic or study in a medical journal.

Help Children Eat Better

The first step in improving your children's diet is to improve your own. You will never succeed in changing their habits to a healthy lifestyle if you are not living one yourself. Follow the recommendations in this book. We are specifically addressing the needs and diets of children over the age of two years. They should consume a healthy balance of food suggested by the food pyramid. Fat should be limited. For instance, after the age of two years, children should not be consuming whole milk and are better off with nonfat milk and nonfat dairy products.

Children learn the type of foods they prefer. We all train our palates. Children can learn to like and prefer the taste of low-fat foods. The reverse is also true: if you have learned to love fat-laden foods, that will be what you prefer. Those tastes can be retrained, but it's easier to start correctly in childhood.

The Family Meal

Research shows that the family meal is an important component in healthy eating for children. A study of 16,000 children, published in the March 2000 issue of *Archives of Family Medicine,* showed that those who had family meals in the evening were more than one-and-a-half times more likely to eat five servings of fruit and vegetables a day. A nutritional analysis showed that they also had a higher intake of fiber, folate, calcium, and vitamins B and E. These children also often had healthier habits throughout the day, when they were out of the home, and consumed less fried food.

HEART POINT

THE FAST FOOD IMPACT:

♦ In 2001, Americans spent $110 billion on fast food.

♦ One-fourth of all Americans visit a fast food restaurant every day.

♦ McDonald's symbol, the golden arches, is more recognized than the †. The average American eats three hamburgers and four orders of French fries every week.

Source: *Fast Food Nation,* by Eric Schlosser

CREATIVE FOOD TIPS:

♦ Cut sandwiches made with whole wheat bread with cookie cutters.
♦ Use nonfat dressing or bean dips with vegetables.
♦ Give kids a selection of two or three healthy snacks to choose from.
♦ For crunch, have air-popped popcorn, carrot sticks, or pretzels.
♦ Use decorative pineapple or other fruit cutouts to liven a meal.

Family meals are wonderful times to teach children good eating habits. It is an opportunity for parents to model a healthy lifestyle for their children. Simply having more healthy food choices available is a significant step forward. Young and picky eaters will have more to choose from. Show young children that you are enjoying healthy foods by making appreciative sounds ("yummmm"). We know it's obvious, but children's curiosity will encourage them to try things that are bringing you pleasure. If children don't want to try what is available, don't order them or nag them to eat it. Also, don't fix a new and special meal for them. If someone did that for you, would you eat the first choice offered? Don't bribe them to eat either. This gets short-term results but really doesn't teach good lifetime eating habits. It's a good idea to eliminate high-fat foods from your house. Bring ice cream and other sweets into your house only for special occasions. Avoid fast food eating; you are teaching your kids to eat high-fat food.

Don't make food an enemy. You want to encourage healthy eating, not an eating disorder. Start to cook with your children at a young age. There are some good, fun cookbooks for cooking with children such as the *Better Homes and Gardens® New Junior Cookbook*. Have fun in the kitchen with your kids and cook healthy recipes together.

Active Children

It is also important to instill children with the pleasure of an active lifestyle. Encourage them to do things they enjoy that get them up off the sofa and away from the computer screen or video games. Expose them to active games and play. Go to the park with younger children, play ball and tennis, and swim with your kids. Let them try ballet, martial arts, and anything else they might enjoy and continue into adulthood. Encourage more physical education in schools and use of the facilities for physical activities at other times. This is very important if your child is overweight and does not want to exercise or be active with all of the kids in the class. This gives the child an opportunity to be active with a group of his or her choosing.

Look for non-school-based programs that promote an active, healthy lifestyle for children. Girls on the Run is just such a program. Started by four-time Hawaii Ironman triathlete Molly Barker, the program, now in more than twenty-five states, encourages girls and their moms to work out a couple of times a week and provides classes on everything from drug and alcohol abuse to other health issues. Along with running, this program now has activities such as rock climbing and backpacking.

CHANGE THE WORLD—
ONE HEART AT A TIME

ELLEN'S STORY

"Changing one heart at a time starts where you live every day. I found out that a coworker's sister was in the hospital. When I asked how her sister was doing, the coworker told me that they had called in a neurologist and cardiologist to run tests. My coworker commented, 'I didn't even know we had heart disease in the family until I told my father what was going on with my sister, and he started to tell me who had died in our family due to heart problems.' She is quite a learned woman, but I couldn't just sit there and let her say that and not comment! I asked her if she knew that she was at risk and told her about my experiences. I explained to her that because heart disease was in my family history, I knew I better be living a healthy lifestyle because heart disease is the largest killer of women, not just men. I didn't push the subject with her, but I wanted her to hear motivation and information from someone else who has heart problems in the family medical history. I talked about the critical need for a healthy diet, exercise, and stress reduction in her life. I hope it made a difference and caused her to think. But just to be sure, I will continue to remind her!"

INFLUENCE FRIENDS AND FAMILY

DARRELL'S STORY

"During my first thallium stress test, the administering cardiologist asked me if I had siblings. After I told him I had a younger sister, he asked me if she was aware of her high risk for heart disease. I decided at that moment that I needed to warn her. I called Linda that night and talked to her about it. She told me she was going for a checkup (the first in years) the next week, so I agreed to send her a letter detailing her risks and include some suggestions of how to approach her doctor and the exam. I'm happy that I did it. I intended the letter as a 'wake-up call' for my sister. Her taking it to her doctor was a good idea. After reading a copy of the letter, her doctor remarked, 'He's very serious about this, isn't he?' Her doctor now takes the risk of heart disease seriously and treats her accordingly."

THE CHANGED LIFESTYLES and testimonials of heart patients and caregivers will be far more motivating to those they love than medical information. Each of you has a responsibility to help educate loved ones who are already at risk and may not be aware of the risk or take it seriously. Reach out to them.

DARRELL'S WARNING LETTER TO HIS SISTER, LINDA

August 27, 1998

Linda,

You have two grandfathers who died, one in his early 50s, the other in his early 60s, from heart attacks, probably as an outgrowth of atherosclerosis. One grandfather had diabetes; your mother probably has diabetes. Your brother, at age 51, has had angioplasty three times since March of 1998, all in the left anterior descending artery: first blockage was 100%, second 95%, and third over 75%. Blockages of from 30 to 50% remain in other areas of that same artery. The surgeon and the noninvasive cardiologist recommend a bypass, if angina symptoms return. Your brother also has slightly elevated blood sugar levels. The diabetes is being aggressively treated using Amaryl (Glimepriride) 4mg per day. His overall cholesterol level is only 108 with a low HDL. The HDL was measured initially at 25 and has now risen to 38. It is also being aggressively treated using Gemfibrozil, 600mg, twice a day. A four-year history of hypertension has been treated with Cardizem cd 240mg per day for most of that time. Diovan 80mg per day was added on 4/8/98.

You have a high risk of developing the same problem. In addition to all the factors above, you went through menopause at an early age. That factor alone raises your risk of a heart attack as high as a man's. I believe you should very aggressively monitor and control hypertension, diabetes, and cholesterol. You should probably have a treadmill stress test, at least to establish a baseline. Then you should change your lifestyle to live on a low fat diet (20% of your calories from fat with little saturated fat). You should lose weight and exercise regularly. The more exercise the better, the more intense the better. (I am now walking four miles every day.) And you should reduce stress levels in your life. (Easy, huh?) In addition, you should take more vitamins and supplements. I'll send the list when you've finished with everything else above.

You should also get and read some books about heart disease for women. You should read the symptoms of angina very carefully. Most doctors DO NOT take heart disease, or even heart attacks, in women seriously!!! I think that over 250,000 women have heart attacks each year. My original primary care doctor misdiagnosed my problem for over five months. His lack of action could easily have killed me. So, know what angina is, how it can feel and insist that every doctor treat those symptoms very seriously. You also should probably start checking on cardiologists. Find a good one, now, maybe even start seeing one now.

That's enough for one day.

Darrell

Bringing About Change

DOCTORS AND NURSES work to diagnose health problems and offer treatment. Hospitals work hard to help sick people become healthy. Health care professionals do not have time to go person to person, promoting a lifestyle that prevents and reverses heart disease. Now that you know what it takes to live heart smart, it is your responsibility to create change. If every heart patient and caregiver who find themselves in a dining situation without heart-smart alternatives would speak out, change would take place.

Think about every event or place where you eat. How can you help bring about change and ensure that you are getting a healthy alternative?

At restaurants

If restaurants offer "lite" menu selections, thank them and order from the healthier choices. Supporting their efforts to offer healthy options will encourage restaurants to keep the items on the menu. Thank the server and manager and then follow up with a letter to the manager and to the corporate headquarters if they have one.

Never hesitate to inquire about a particular menu item. If the restaurant truly believes in customer service and wants your business, staff will not mind answering questions. Find out how foods are cooked. "Grilled" sounds great until you discover the meat was drenched with melted butter and wine first. Ask if the chef can cook your selection without butter or vegetable oil. Have high-fat toppings left off. Ask for low-fat salad dressing or at least ask for your dressing on the side so you can monitor how much you use.

On airplanes

If your scheduled flight includes a meal, call ahead to prearrange a healthier meal option. Many airlines offer alternatives. When you are served your meal, if it's really a healthy alternative, make sure you tell the flight attendant how much you appreciate the opportunity to choose. If the meal is not extremely healthy, write a letter to the customer service department of the airline and offer suggestions on healthier in-flight meals. If there is no meal on your flight or no choices, take along a healthy alternative. Think about carrying fruit for snacks on all trips.

At the office or business events

Many large corporations have their own cafeterias. If the cafeteria or snack shop at your office doesn't offer healthy alternatives, start making suggestions. Find out who runs the cafeteria and talk to the manager. If that doesn't get the ball rolling, go to your human resources department. Discuss the human and corporate costs of heart disease and propose a wellness program.

Be the one who asks what will be served at the annual sales reception or banquet and strongly suggest a healthy alternative. Call ahead to ask for something healthy. In addition, check the menu for any office party. If healthy options are not included, volunteer to bring something. Fresh fruit or vegetables are always a good option.

Finally, when someone is making a fast food "run" for lunch and you are asked if you want to place an order, decline.

At church

In order to reach out to the growing needs of families, many churches offer meals before regular activities. In an effort to tickle the taste buds of both children and adults, the menu may be missing healthy options. Read cookbooks and magazines that offer healthier, low-fat recipes and collect these for the person in charge of food preparation. Take note of the number of heart disease patients you know in your congregation who would live longer if they ate healthier. Guilt works well in a religious setting!

With friends and relatives

It's one thing to "make waves" with a national airline, but it can get tricky and sticky to bring up the subject of healthier menus with family and friends. However, if they are truly your friends and if they genuinely care about you, they will be more than glad to find healthy selections to serve. This is particularly true after you have had a bypass or heart attack. Use that experience to educate everyone. Perhaps you can offer to help with the meal and bring the healthy options yourself for the first time or two. They can only start to understand how important healthy eating is to you and your family only when you raise the issue with them. Do it politely, but firmly. Family traditions and holidays are often saturated with unhealthy food choices. It's time for you to start some new ones. When the family or friends come to your house, surprise them with healthy foods that taste great. Set the example for them to follow.

REACHING OUT TO TOUCH SOMEONE

DARRELL'S STORY

"During a television segment to promote one of my gardening books, I had an opportunity to start changing one heart at a time. Before my segment, the show was doing a remote broadcast from a local restaurant. The camera panned across plates of fried catfish, fried chicken, and huge platters of barbecued ribs. Most of the people in the studio were practically drooling. The host turned to me and asked if I loved ribs. I told him that I loved them and used to eat them. I quickly explained about my heart disease, angioplasties, triple bypass, and my new lifestyle. His mouth dropped open in surprise. He couldn't believe it. I further explained that my healthy lifestyle, before the diagnosis, probably saved my life, and that I must have inherited some bad genes. He began to tell me about his family history of heart disease and commented further that his doctor had not even given him an EKG during his last physical.

"We went on the air and I did my segment. I had to leave the studio as they finished the show, so we did not get to talk anymore. After returning to New York, I sent him a letter summarizing the risk factors and suggesting steps to help him take charge of his heart. I sincerely hope he has!"

Think about sending a letter like this one to someone at risk:

Dear _____ :

The reason for this note is my concern for you and your risk of heart disease. I saw your concern and surprise when you heard about my experience. Yes, I was a person who had improved my lifestyle, resulting in a good diet and a high level of exercise (by average standards.) In spite of that, I did develop blockages in my arteries that were badly misdiagnosed for about five months. Ten days after my first visit to a cardiologist I had my first angioplasty. In the next five months, I had two more, and then I had a triple bypass.

Between the first hospitalization and the bypass, I changed from a passive consumer of medical care to being a major decision maker and force in my treatment and care. I found that this was a major step in what my surgeon described as a "spectacular recovery."

Though I do not want to pry, I already am aware of a few things that give me concern about your medical history and want to make some comments for you to think about. I know you have a strong family history of heart disease (you told me that), you are male, and are near or over fifty. These are substantial risk factors for heart disease that you cannot change. Other factors can and will add to that risk. They are:

High blood pressure—If not controlled, it makes your heart work harder and accelerates atherosclerosis (hardening of the arteries).

High blood cholesterol—If your total cholesterol is high it means that your LDL (low-density lipoprotein), which is the "lousy" cholesterol, is high. If your HDL, your "healthy" cholesterol, is low (under 40), you also have a problem. There is some controversy about what the numbers should be, but an aggressive approach would aim for LDL of 130 or less. (Once heart disease has been diagnosed, the goal is lower; my target is to maintain LDL at less than 100.) Cholesterol levels can be controlled by eating a low-fat diet, getting regular exercise, and in some cases, taking medication.

Diabetes—This is a significant heart disease risk factor. Your cardiovascular risk increases even more if you have both high blood pres-

sure and diabetes. The chance of coronary heart disease and heart attack is increased two to six times in diabetics. The official definition of diabetes (or the threshold) has been changed to suggest treatment much earlier. My blood sugar levels were only slightly elevated and were untreated by my former doctor. My current endocrinologist calls my type of diabetes the insidious kind. Any abnormalities should be aggressively treated.

Stress—Stress may be a much larger contributing factor than previously believed. Most of us are much too tense and have many things that create stress in day-to-day life. I know you lead a stressful life. I took a stress management course and exercise. I still need to do more about stress.

Diet and exercise—These can be risk factors or a positive. Most Americans eat too much and eat the wrong things (high in fat and sugar, low in fiber). Most Americans do not exercise enough. Research shows (published studies in JAMA) that blockages in arteries can be reversed by eating a diet low in fat, getting enough exercise, and reducing stress. Dr. Dean Ornish's work suggests a diet that has only 10 percent of the calories from fat. This is extreme, virtually a vegetarian diet with no fish or poultry and no added fat of any kind. I am striving for about 15 percent fat and have given up all red meat and eat only a little fish or chicken. Research shows that if you burn about 2,500 calories a week from exercise you may reverse blockages. I try to walk four miles a day at a fast pace, about 120 heartbeats per minute.

Smoking—don't.

Lose weight.

Taking charge—Maybe the most important thing I did was to educate myself and take charge of my health. I started educating myself to stay alive. The information above is just a beginning; you need to learn more. It seems like you and your siblings are all at high risk. I was very surprised that your doctor did not do an electrocardiogram during your checkup. It is not a very effective diagnostic tool, but I think he should have done a "baseline" one. (Even when I was having angina pain, my EKG results were normal because my heart was not stressed at that moment.)

As a first step, I would find an excellent cardiologist. Check your health plan to find out who you can go to and research and select a good one; then get a referral from your doctor to the cardiologist you have chosen. If your doctor doesn't want to take this seriously or give you the referral, change doctors. I think you are more concerned about this than he is, so you need to take charge. Doctors don't know everything—my original doctor almost killed me. Or, if you have to pay for some of those tests out of your own pocket, I would do it.

You also should monitor your body and how you feel. The single most important diagnostic tool doctors have is listening to you. You need to be particularly aware of any chest pain or pressure as well as pains— often spreading and usually symmetrical in your arms, shoulders, or hands—that occur during exertion. Don't deny symptoms; get them checked out. Symptoms of angina and even heart attack are not always the same for everyone. Read more about both of those and learn to monitor your own body.

The above is only a rough outline of some of the risk factors and some of the things I do to keep myself alive. I hope this starts you thinking and on the road to learning more and keeping yourself healthy. If you have any questions about any of this give me a call.

Sincerely yours,

Who can you influence? With whom can you share your story? You never know the impact you might be having on someone else's life or the life of someone he or she loves. Whether you are on a plane, on a bus, or in the next cubicle at work, encourage people to take control of their health. You may be the life that saves a life. It is not enough to save your own life. The people in your sphere of influence need the knowledge and understanding you have gained through having heart disease and reading this book. It is hard for someone to ignore an urgent message from a friend or loved one. Talk to those close to you about heart disease with a sense of urgency. Make it your own personal mandate. Share it from the heart.

BIBLIOGRAPHY

STAR POINT ONE: TAKE CHARGE OF YOUR HEART

Charlesworth, Edward, Ph.D., and Ronald G. Nathan, Ph.D. *Stress Management: A Comprehensive Guide to Your Well-Being.* New York: Ballantine Books, 1984.

Friedman, Meyer, M.D. *Type A Behavior and Your Heart.* New York: Alfred A. Knopf, 1974.

Kwiterovich, Peter O., Jr., M.D. *The Johns Hopkins Complete Guide to Preventing and Reversing Heart Disease.* Rocklin, CA: Prima Health, 1998.

Levin, Rhoda F., M.S.W. *Heartmates: A Guide for the Spouse and Family of the Heart Patient.* Rev. ed. Minneapolis, MN: Minerva Press, 1994.

McFarlane, Rodger, and Philip Bashe. *The Complete Bedside Companion.* New York: Simon & Schuster, 1998.

McIlwain, Harris, M.D., and Debra Bruce. *My Parent, My Turn.* Nashville, TN: Broadman & Holman, 1995.

National Institute of Diabetes and Digestive and Kidney Diseases. "Statistics Related to Overweight and Obesity." NIH Pub. No. 96-4158, July 1996; e-text posted: 12 February 1998, updated: June 2000, www.niddk.nih.gov/health/nutrit/pubs/statobes.htm.

"Obesity Defined," *New York Times,* January 12, 1997.

Ornish, Dean, M.D. *Dr. Dean Ornish's Program for Reversing Heart Disease.* New York: Random House, 1990.

Piscatella, Joseph C. *Choices for a Healthy Heart.* New York: Workman Publishing, 1987.

Ramachandran, S. Vasan, M.D., et al. "Impact of High-Normal Blood Pressure on Cardiovascular Disease" (research from the Framingham Heart Study), *New England Journal of Medicine* 345 (18): 1291–1297, 2001.

"Smoking and Health: A Report of the Surgeon General." DHEW Pub. No. (PHS) 79-50066. Washington, D.C., 1979.

"Type 2 Diabetes in Children and Adolescents, Consensus Statement American Diabetes Association," *Diabetes Care* 22(12):381–399, 2000.

Vartiainen, Ilmari, M.D., and Karl Kanerva, M.D. *Annals of Internal Medicine* 536:748–758, 1947.

Whitaker, Julian M., M.D. *Reversing Heart Disease.* New York: Warner Books, Inc., 1985.

STAR POINT TWO: EDUCATE YOURSELF

Castelli, William P., et al. "Incidence of Coronary Heart Disease and Lipoprotein Cholesterol Levels—The Framingham Study," *JAMA* 256:2835–2838, 1986.

Clayman, Charles B., medical editor. *Your Heart.* Pleasantville, NY/Montreal: The American Medical Association, 1989.

The National Geographic Society, *The Incredible Machine.* Washington, D.C., 1994.

Public Citizen Health Research Group. *20,125 Questionable Doctors Disciplined by State and Federal Governments* (CD-ROM). Washington, D.C., 2000.

Rob, Caroline, R.N. *The Caregiver's Guide.* Boston: Houghton Mifflin, 1991.

Vasan, Ramachandran S., M.D. "Impact of High-Normal Blood Pressure on the Risk of Cardiovascular Disease," *New England Journal of Medicine* 345(18):1291–1297, 2001.

STAR POINT THREE: LEAD YOUR TEAM

Brody, Jane, E. "Now, Choices in Heart Bypass Surgery," e-text, Personal Health Archive, *The New York Times,* March 6, 2001.

Bush, D. E., R. D. Ziegelstein, et al. "Even Minimal Symptoms of Depression Increase Mortality Risk After Acute Myocardial Infarction," *Am J Cardiol* 5:337–341, 2001.

"Co-Occurrence of Depression and Heart Disease," fact sheet, National Institute of Mental Health (NIMH), Updated: June 1, 1999.

Faughun, Susan. *Half Empty, Half Full: Understanding the Psychological Roots of Optimism.* New York: Harcourt, 2001.

Hochman, Gloria. *Heart Bypass.* New York: St. Martin's Press, 1982.

Horowitz, Lawrence C., M.D. *Taking Charge of Your Medical Fate.* New York: Random House, 1988.

Inlander, Charles B. *Good Operations Bad Operations.* New York: Viking, 1993.

Luchi, R. J., et al. "Comparison of Medical and Surgical treatment for Unstable Angina Pectoris," *New England Journal of Medicine* 316(16):977–984, 1987.

Nallamothu, B. K., et al. "The Role of Hospital Volume in Coronary Artery Bypass Grafting: Is More Always Better?" *J Am Coll Cardiol* 38(7):1931–1933, 2001.

"A Randomized Trial of Coronary Artery Bypass Surgery: Quality of Life in Patients Randomly Assigned to Treatment Groups," *Circulation* 68(5):951–960, 1983.

Roizen, Michael F., M.D. *Real Age: Are You as Young as You Can Be?* New York: Cliff Street Book, HarperCollins, 1999.

Romaine, Deborah S., and Dawn E. DeWitt, M.D. *The Complete Idiot's Guide to a Happy, Healthy Heart.* New York: Alpha Books, 1998.

Selnes, Ola A., Ph.D., and Guy M. McKhann, M.D. "Coronary-Artery Bypass Surgery and the Brain," *New England Journal of Medicine* 344(6):451–452, 2001.

Whitaker, Julian, M.D. *Is Heart Surgery Necessary?* Washington, D.C.: Regnery Publishing, 1995.

STAR POINT FOUR: MANAGE YOUR TREATMENT

Brown, B. Greg, et al. "Simvastatin and Niacin, Antioxidant Vitamins, or the Combination for the Prevention of Coronary Disease," *New England Journal of Medicine* 5(48):1583–1592, 2001.

Cheng, Judy, W. M. "Patient-Reported Adherence to Guidelines of the Sixth Joint National Committee on Prevention, Detection, Evaluation, and Treatment of High Blood Pressure," *Pharmacotherapy* 21(7):828–841, 2001.

Cohen, Jay Sylvan, M.D. *Make Your Medicine Safe: How to Prevent Side Effects from the Drugs You Take.* New York: Avon Books, 1998

Graedon, Joe, and Teresa Graedon, Ph.D. *The People's Guide to Deadly Drug Interactions: How to Protect Yourself from Life-Threatening Drug/Drug, Drug/Food, Drug/Vitamin Combinations.* New York: St. Martin's Press, 1995.

Gum, Patricia A., M.D., et al. "Aspirin Use and All-Cause Mortality Among Patients Being Evaluated for Known or Suspected Coronary Artery Disease," *JAMA* 286 (10):1187–1194, 2001.

How to Find the Best Doctors for You and Your Family: New York Metro Area. New York: Castle Connolly Medical Ltd., 1994.

Institute for Safe Medication Practices. "Request a Brown Bag Checkup," May 16, 2002, www.ismp.org/consumer/brownbag.html.

Knudtson, Merril L., et al. "Chelation Therapy for Ischemic Heart Disease," *JAMA* 287(4):481–486, 2002.

Lawson, William E., et al. "Efficacy of Enhanced External Counterpulsation in the Treatment of Angina Pectoris," *Am J Cardiol* 70:859–862, 1992.

———. "Three Year Sustained Benefit from Enhanced External Counterpulsation in Chronic Angina Pectoris," *Am J Cardiol* 75:840–841, 1995.

Morton, Ian, Ph.D., and Judith Hall, Ph.D. *The Avery Complete Guide to Medicines.* New York: Avery, 2001.

Saint Francis Hospital, The Nutrition, Pharmacy, and Nursing Departments, "Drug & Food Interaction Reference Guide," Form 80301. Roslyn, NY: 1997.

Tyberg, Theodore, M.D., and Kenneth Rothaus, M.D. *Hospital Smarts.* New York: Hearst Books, 1995.

U.S. Food and Drug Administration/Center for Drug Evaluation and Research, "Medication Question Guide," e-text, www.fda.gov.cder.consumerinfo/ question_guide.htm., last update October 9, 2001.

Wolfe, Sidney M. (ed.), Larry D. Sasich, and Rose-Ellen Hope. *Worst Pills, Best Pills: A Consumer's Guide to Avoiding Drug-Induced Death or Illness.* Washington, D.C.: Public Citizen Research Group, 1999.

"Vice President Gore Unveils New Safety Labeling Requirements for Over-The-Counter Medications," White House Press Release, Office of the Vice President, March 11, 1999.

STAR POINT FIVE: LIVE HEART SMART

CONTROLLING STRESS

Allen, K., B. E. Shykoff, and J. L. Izzo, Jr. "Pet Ownership, but Not ACE Inhibitor Therapy, Blunts Home Blood Pressure Responses to Mental Stress," *Hypertension* 38(4):815–820, 2001.

Benson, Herbert, M.D. *The Relaxation Response.* New York: Avon Books, 1976.

Blumenthal, James, et al. "Stress Management and Exercise Training in Cardiac Patients with Myocardial Ischemia," *Archives of Internal Medicine* 157:2213–2223, 1997.

Cousins, Norman. *The Healing Heart, Antidotes to Panic and Helplessness.* New York: W.W. Norton & Company, 1983.

Gates, Anita. "Pitter-Patter of Paws is Time-Tested Remedy," e-text, *The New York Times,* July 24, 2001.

Hochman, Gloria. *Heart Bypass.* New York: St. Martin's Press, 1982.

"Laughter and Medicine: How Humor Can Help You Heal," Mayoclinic.com, posted September 28, 2001.

Lee Williams, J. E., et al. "Anger Proneness Predicts Coronary Heart Disease Risk," *Circulation* 101(17):2034–2039, 2000.

Levin, Rhoda F., M.S.W. *Heartmates: A Guide for the Spouse and Family of the Heart Patient.* Minneapolis, MN: Minerva Press, 1994.

Miller, Lyle H., Ph.D., and Alma Dell Smith, Ph.D., with Larry Rothstein, Ed.D. *The Stress Solution.* New York: Pocket Books, 1993.

Newman, Judith. "C'Mon Get Happy," *Health* 131(146):131–139, 193–194, 2000.

Ornish, Dean, M.D. *Stress, Diet, & Your Heart.* New York: Signet, 1984.

"Stress," *Newsweek,* June 14:58–68, 1999.

"Today: News and Events," website for Loma Linda Adventist University Health Science Center, posted September 20, 2001, Lee S. Berk, DrPH paper, "The Anticipation of a Laughter Eustress Event Modulates Mood States Prior to the Actual Humor Experience." Presented and published at the Society of Neuroscience annual meeting on November 10–15, 2001. www.llu.edu/news/today/sept2001/sm.html.

Vollmer, W. M., et al. "Effects of Diet and Sodium Intake on Blood Pressure: Subgroup Analysis of the DASH-Sodium Trial," *Annals of Internal Medicine* 135(12):1019–1028, 2001.

EAT TO LIVE

Brazzano, Lydia A., et al. "Legume Consumption and Risk of Coronary Heart Disease in US Men and Women," *Archives of Internal Medicine* 161:2573–2578, 2001.

Brody, Jane E. "Personal Health: Added Sugars Are Taking a Toll," *The New York Times,* September 12, 2000.

Brody, Jane E., and the reporters of *The New York Times, The New York Times Book of Health.* New York: Times Books, 1997.

Claiborne, Craig, with Pierre Franey. *Craig Claiborne's Gourmet Diet.* New York: Ballantine Books, 1980.

Cooper, Kenneth, M.D. *Dr. Kenneth H. Cooper's Antioxidant Revolution.* Nashville, TN: Thomas Nelson Publishers, 1994.

Cooper, R., et al. "Seventh-Day Adventist Adolescents–Life-Style Patterns and Cardiovas-cular Risk Factors," *Western Journal of Medicine* 140: 1984.

Davis, Adelle. *Let's Cook It Right.* New York: Signet, The New American Library, Inc., 1970.

DeBakey, Michael E., M.D., Antonio M. Gotto, M.D., et al. *The New Living Heart Diet.* New York: Simon & Schuster, 1996.

Kato, H., et al. "Epidemiologic Studies of Coronary Heart Disease and Stroke in Japanese Men Living in Japan, Hawaii, and California. Serum Lipids and Diet," *American Journal of Epidemiology* 97(6):372–385, 1973.

Keys, A. "Coronary Heart Disease in Seven Countries," *Circulation* 41, 1970.

Keys, Ancel, M.D. "Lessons from Serum Cholesterol Studies in Japan, Hawaii and Los Angeles," *Annals of Internal Medicine* 48:83, 1958.

Mateljan, George. *Baking Without Fat.* Irwindale, CA: Health Valley Foods, 1994.

Mayfield, Eleanor. "A Consumer's Guide to Fat," Pub. No. (FDA) 99-2286. Washington, D.C.: U.S. Food and Drug Administration, FDA Consumer, May 1994: revised November 1994, January 1996, and January 1999.

Ornish, Dean, M.D. *Eat More, Weigh Less.* New York: Harper Collins, 1993.

Spear, Ruth. *Low Fat & Loving It.* New York: Warner Books, Inc., 1991.

"Statistics Related to Overweight and Obesity," NIH Publication No. 96-4158, July 1996, e-text posted: 12 February 1998, updated: June 2000.

Sturm, R., and K. B. Wells. "Does Obesity Contribute as much to Morbidity as Poverty or Smoking?" *Public Health* 115:229–235, 2001.

Tracey, Elizabeth. "Removing Trans Fats from Foods Could Save Lives, FDA Says," WebMD Medical News, posted June 6, 2000, www.my.webmd.com/content/article/1728.58208.

Volmer, W. M., et al. "Special Diets Reduce Blood Pressure," *Annals of Internal Medicine* 135(12):1018–1028, 2001.

QUIT SMOKING

Esopenko, Gerald. *Stop Smoking Made Easy.* Deerfield Beach, FL: Made E-Z Products, Inc., 2000.

Friedman, G. D., et al. "Mortality in Cigarette Smokers and Quitters," *New England Journal of Medicine* 304(23):1400–1410, 1981.

CLEARING THE AIR:
HOW TO QUIT SMOKING . . . AND QUIT FOR KEEPS

National Cancer Institute, div. of National Institutes of Health (NIH)

EXERCISE

Armstrong, M. L., et al. "Regression of Coronary Atherosclerosis in Rhesus Monkeys," *Circulatory Research,* 1959.

Fletcher, Gerald F., M.D., et al. "Statement on Exercise: Benefits and Recommendations for Physical Activity Programs for All Americans," *Circulation* 94:857–862, 1996.

Hambrecht, R., and J. Niebauer, et al. "Various Intensities of Leisure Time Physical Activity in Patients with Coronary Artery Disease: Effects on Cardio Respiratory Fitness and Progression of Coronary Atherosclerotic Lesions," *J Am Coll Cardiol* 22:468–477, 1993.

"Intensive Exercise Improves Body's Ability to Process Blood Sugars," Duke University Medical Center website, accessed February 14, 2002, www.dukenews.duke.edu/med/sugar.htm.

Institute for the Study of Aging and International Longevity Center—USA. "Achieving and Maintaining Cognitive Vitality with Aging" (Workshop Report). New York: Author, 2001.

Lane, Laura. "Walking Reduces Women's Heart-Attack Risk," CNN website (with WebMD.com), August 25, 1999, www.cnn.com/HEALTH/heart/9908/25/heart.ecise/.

Paffenbarger, R. S., Jr. "Contributions of Epidemiology to Exercise Science and Cardiovascular Health," *Med. Sci. Sports Exerc.* 20(5):426–438, 1988.

Paffenbarger, R. S., Jr., R.T. Hyde, et al. "Physical Activity, All-Cause Mortality, and Longevity of College Alumni," *New England Journal of Medicine* 314:605–613, 1986.

"Warning: Too Much TV Is Hazardous to Your Health," Turn Off TV Fact Sheet, 2001, www.turnofftv.org/images/facts&figs/factsheets/hazardous.pdf.

CARDIAC REHABILITATION

Center for Disease Control and Prevention. *Cardiovascular Disease Risk Factors and Preventive Practices Among Adults—United States, 1994: A Behavioral Risk Factor Atlas, Surveillance Summaries.* Atlanta, 1998.

Giambrone, Laurie, M.A. (sr. exercise physiologist). "Cardiac Fitness & Rehabilitation at St. Francis Hospital," undated report.

U.S. Department of Health and Human Services, Agency for Health Care Policy and Research. "Recovering from Heart Problems Through Cardiac Rehabilitation," AHCPR Publication No. 96-0674. Washington, D.C.: October 1995.

STAR POINT SIX: EMBRACE SUPPORT

Anderson, Greg. *The 22 (Non-Negotiable) Laws of Wellness.* New York: Harper Collins, 1995.

Berkman L. F., L. Leo-Summers, and R. I. Horwitz. "Emotional Support and Survival after Myocardial Infarction: A Prospective, Population-Based Study of the Elderly," *Annals of Internal Medicine* 117(12):1003–1009, 1992.

Berkman, Lisa F., and Lester Breslow. *Health and Ways of Living: The Alameda County Study.* New York: Oxford University Press, 1983.

Bernardi, Luciano, M.D., "Effect of Rosary Prayer and Yoga Mantas on Autonomic cardiovascular Rhythms: Comparative Study," *British Medical Journal* 323:1446–1449, 2001.

"Coping as You Care," *Health* 134(173):134–138, 172–177, 2000.

Cortis, Bruno, M.D. *Heart & Soul: A Psychological and Spiritual Guide to Preventing and Healing Heart Disease.* New York: Villard Books, 1995.

Cousins, Norman. *Anatomy of an Illness.* New York: W.W. Norton, 1979.

Doka, Kenneth J. *Living with Life-Threatening Illness: A Guide for Patients, Their Families, & Caregivers.* New York: Lexington Books, 1993.

Dreher, Henry, M.D. *Immune Power Personalty: 7 Traits You Can Develop to Stay Healthy.* New York: EP Dutton, 1995.

Hallqvist, Johan, et al. "Socioeconomic Difference in Risk for Myocardial Infarction 1971–94 Among Men and Women in Sweden," *International Journal of Epidemiology* 27:410–415, 1998.

Ivker, Rovert, M.D., and Edward Zorensky. *Thriving: The Complete Mind/Body Guide for Optimal Health and Fitness for Men.* New York: Random House, 1997.

Koenig, H. G., and D. B. Larson. "Use of Hospital Services, Religious Attendance, and Religious Affiliation," *Southern Medical Journal* 91(10):925–932, 1998.

Martin, Paul R. *The Healing Mind: The Vital Links Between Brain and Behavior, Immunity and Disease.* New York: St. Martins Press, 1998.

Moody, Raymond A., Jr., M.D. *Laugh After Laugh: The Healing Power of Humor.* Jacksonville, FL: Headwaters Press, 1978.

National Family Caregiver Association, "Member Survey 1997: A Profile of Caregivers," www.nfcacares.org/survey.html., May 15, 2002.

Ornstein, Robert, and David Sobel. *The Healing Brain: Breakthrough Discoveries About How the Brain Keeps Us Healthy.* New York: Simon & Schuster, 1987.

Orth-Gomer, K., and J. V. Johnson. "Social Network Interaction and Mortality: A Six-Year Follow-up Study of a Random Sample of the Swedish Population," *Journal of Chronic Diseases* 40:949–957, 1987.

Padus, Emrika, and the editors of *Prevention* magazine. T*he Complete Guide to Your Emotions & Your Health: New Dimensions in Mind/Body Healing.* Emmaus, PA: Rodale Press, Inc., 1986.

Seligman, Martin E.P., Ph.D. *Learned Optimism: How to Change Your Mind and Your Life.* New York: Pocket Books, 1990.

Siegel, Bernie S., M.D. *Love, Medicine, & Miracles: Lessons Learned about Self-Healing from a Surgeon's Experience with Exceptional Patients.* New York, Harper & Row, 1986.

Strohl, Lydia. "Why Do Doctors Now Believe Faith Heals?" *Reader's Digest* 109(15):64–66, 2001.

CHAPTER SEVEN: WOMEN AND HEART DISEASE

American Heart Association, "American Heart Association Science Advisory: Hormone Replacement Therapy and Cardiovascular Disease," American Heart Association website, http://216.185.112.5/presenter.jhtml?identifier=10975, posted July 1, 2001.

————. "Women, Heart Disease and Stroke Survey Highlights & Comparisons 2000," American Heart Association website, http://216.185.112.5/presenter.jhtml?identifier=10382.

Hankinson, Susan E., R.N., Sc.D., Graham A. Colditz, M.D., et al. (eds.), *Healthy Women, Healthy Lives: A Guide to Preventing Disease, from the Landmark Nurses' Health Study.* New York: Simon & Schuster, 2001.

Helfant, Richard H., M.D. *The Women's Guide to Fighting Heart Disease.* New York: The Berkley Publishing Group, A Perigee Book, 1993.

Kayplan, Jan. "Stress and Heart Disease in Women," *The Green Journal* 99: 381–388, 2002.

Kra, Siegfried J. *What Every Woman Must Know About Heart Disease.* New York: Warner Books, Inc., 1996.

Lowen, Alexander, M.D. *Love, Sex, and Your Heart.* New York: Macmillan Publishing Company, 1988.

Marrugat, Jaume, M.D., et al. "Mortality Differences Between Men and Women Following First Myocardial Infarction," *JAMA* 280:1405–1409, 1998.

National Institutes of Health. "Facts about Heart Disease and Women: Are You at Risk?" NIH Publication No. 98-3654. Bethesda, MD: August 1998 (rev.).

———. *The Sixth Report of the Joint National Committee on Detection, Evaluation, and Treatment of High Blood Pressure.* Bethesda, MD: National Heart, Lung, and Blood Institute (NHLBI), 1997.

Ojeda, Linda, Ph.D. *Her Healthy Heart: A Woman's Guide to Preventing and Reversing Heart Disease Naturally.* Alameda, CA: Hunter House Inc., 1998.

"Physical Activity and Health: A Report of the Surgeon General," Stock number AD-A329-047/5INT www.surgeongeneral.gov, and www.cdc.gov/nccdphp/sgr/sgr.htm, last update November 17, 1999.

Pratt, Laura A., et al. "Depression, Psychotropic Medication, and Risk of Myocardial Infarction," *Circulation* 94:3123–3129, 1996.

Singh, Mantosh. *Strong Women, Weak Hearts: Women and Heart Disease A Personal Perspective.* New York: International Science Publisher, 1993.

Smith, Nancy F. "Town and Country's Comprehensive Guide to the Healthy Heart," *Town & Country* 109(116):110–116, 1999.

"What's Different About Heart Disease in Women?" with Debra J. Judelson, M.D., WebMD Live Chat Transcript, http://my.webmd.com/content/asset/ chat_transcript.506584, May 12, 1999.

CHAPTER EIGHT: TEACH YOUR CHILDREN WELL

Better Homes and Gardens® New Jr. Cookbook. Des Moines, IA: Meredith Corporation, 1997.

Gillman, Matthew, R., M.D., et al. "Family Diet and Dinner Quality Among Older Adolescents," *Archives of Family Medicine,* March 2000.

Schlosser, Eric. *Fast Food Nation.* New York: Perennial, 2002.

"The Surgeon General's Call to Action to Prevent and Decrease Overweight and Obesity," Surgeon General's webiste, www.surgeongeneral.gov.topics/obesity/.

"Type 2 Diabetes in Children and Adolescents" (Consensus Statement American Diabetes Association), *Diabetes Care* 22(12):381–398, 2000.

RESOURCES

Getting More Help

ALTERNATIVE MEDICINE

Vicus
Alternative medicine source and links.
www.Vicus.com

DIABETES

American Diabetes Association
1660 Duke Street Alexandria, VA 22314
800-232-3472 or 703-549-1500
www.diabetes.org

National Diabetes Information Clearinghouse (NDIC)
Box NDIC
9000 Rockville Pike
Bethesda, MD 20892
301-468-2162
Information to patients and families about diabetes.
www.niddk.nih.gov/health/diabetes/ndic

DIET AND OBESITY

American Dietetic Association
Consumer Education Team
216 West Jackson Boulevard
Chicago, IL 60606
(Send self-addressed stamped envelope for nutrition fact sheets)

800-877-1600, ext. 5000, for other publications
800-366-1655 for recorded food/nutrition messages
www.eatright.com

American Obesity Association
1250 24th Street, NW, Suite 300
Washington, DC 20037
800-98-OBESE

American Society of Bariatric Physicians (ASBP)
5600 South Quebec Street, Suite 109-A
Englewood, CO 80111 USA
303-779-4833 or 303-770-2526
Fax: 303-779-4834
E-mail: bariatric@asbp.org

The Council on Size and Weight Discrimination
P.O. Box 305
Mt. Marion, NY 12456
(Send self-addressed stamped envelope)

Federal Trade Commission
Consumer Response Center
600 Pennsylvania Avenue, NW
Washington, DC 20580
202-FTC-HELP

National Institute of Diabetes and Digestive and Kidney Diseases
31 Center Drive
Bethesda, MD 20892
301-496-3583

North American Association for the Study of Obesity
8630 Fenton Street
Silver Spring, MD 20910

Weight-Control Information Network
1 Win Way
Bethesda, MD 20892-3665
202-828-1025 or 1-877-946-4627
Fax: 202-828-1028
E-mail: win@info.niddk.nih.gov
www.niddk.nih.gov/health/nutrit/pubs/choose.htm

DOCTORS AND HOSPITALS

American Board of Medical Specialties
Searchable database of board certified specialties: www.certifieddoctor.org

American Medical Association
Searchable database of 690,000 physicians: www.ama-assn.org/

Best Doctors
Finding the best doctors: www.bestdoctors.com

Lerner's Consumer Guide to Healthcare
Healthcare advocates and information source: www.lernerhealth.com

NY State Dept. of Health
List of disciplined doctors (click on information for consumers then Professional
Misconduct): www.health.state.ny.us
(Check your state's website, more information is available all the time.)

WellnessWeb
Information about communicating with doctors: www.wellweb.com

GENERAL HEALTH

Consumer Information Center
Pueblo, CO 81009
Catalog of free or low-cost booklets on many health-related topics.

Food and Drug Administration (FDA)
Office of Consumer Affairs, HFE-88
5600 Fishers Lane
Rockville, MD 20857
301-443-3170
www.fda.gov

HealthAtoZ
Interactive disease information.
www.HealthAtoZ.com

Healthfinder
A health portal (government-run), connections to many good sites.
www.healthfinder.gov

HealthTalk Interactive
Information for people with serious illnesses.
www.healthtalk.com

Intelihealth
Health information in understandable terms from Harvard Medical School.
www.intelihealth.com

National Institutes of Health
Government-based information all health issues.
www.nhlbi.nih.gov

National Heart, Lung, and Blood Institute (NHLBI) Information Center
NHLBI Information Center
P.O. Box 30105
Bethesda, MD 20824-0105
301-251-1222
Information about cholesterol, smoking, obesity, high blood pressure, and heart disease.
www.nhlbi.nih.gov/nhlbi/nhlbi.htm

National Library of Medicine
U.S. Department of Health and Human Services
Building 38A, Room 3N-305
8600 Rockville Pike
Bethesda, MD 20894
301-496-1131
Free directory of health-related organizations with 800 numbers.

Quackwatch
Health scams and myths.
www.quackwatch.com

HEART DISEASE

ABOUT.COM
Sections on heart disease, diabetes, walking, and healthy recipes.
www.about.com

American Heart Association
National Center
7320 Greenville Avenue
Dallas, TX 75231
214-373-6300
www.americanheart.org

Cholesterol, Genetics, and Heart Disease Institute
For physicians but much readable information.
www.heartdisease.org

Clinical Trials Center
Clinical trials recruiting patients, some heart disease related.
www.centerwatch.com/LISTING.HTML

Heartcenteronline
www.heartcenteronline.com/myheartdr/home/index.cfm

Heart Information Network
Independent website with wide range of information for heart patients.
www.heartinfo.com

Infinity Heart Institute interactive; allows you to ask doctor questions.
www.infinityheart.com/askdoc.html

Surviving with Heart
Authors' website; updates on heart disease
www.survivingwithheart.com

INSURANCE (HEALTH)

Georgetown University's Institute for Health Care Research
In-depth information on your health insurance rights for all fifty states.
www.healthinsuranceinfo.net

MEDICINES AND SUPPLEMENTS

American Society of Health System Pharmacists
Side effects and optimal use of prescription and over-the-counter drugs.
www.safemedication.com

DrugChecker.com
A drug checker function at Dr.Koop.com that allows searching for interactions.
www.drugchecker.com

Institute for Safe Medication Practices
1800 Byberry Road, Suite 810
Huntingdon Valley, PA 19006
www.ismp.org

Medscape Druginfo Database
Drug Search 2000 is a powerful drug information search tool.
www.promini.medscape.com/drugdb/search.asp

Medline plus
A searchable database including drugs.
www.nlm.nih.gov/medlineplus/

National Institutes of Health
Database for recent research on supplements.
www.odp.od.nih.gov/ods/databases/ibids.html

SENIOR ADVOCATES

American Association of Retired Persons
AARP
P.O. Box 199
Long Beach, CA 90801
800-424-3410
www.AARP.org

National Association of Area Agencies on Aging
1112 16th Street NW, Suite 100
Washington, DC 20036
To get the number of the nearest agency in your area, call 800-555-1212.

SMOKING; RESOURCES FOR STOPPING

American Cancer Society
1599 Clifton Road NE
Atlanta, GA 30329
800-ACS-2345; 404-320-3333
Information on smoking and how to stop.
www.cancer.org

American Lung Association
1740 Broadway
New York, NY 10019-4374
212-315-8700

STRESS

American Institute of Stress
124 Park Avenue
Yonkers, NY 10703
Information on managing stress.
1-800-24-RELAX (247-3529)

STROKE

National Stroke Association
96 Inverness Drive E, Suite I
Englewood, CO 80112-5112
303-649-9299
Stroke prevention, treatment, rehabilitation, research, and support for survivors and families.
www.stroke.org

SUPPORT GROUPS

Mended Hearts, Inc.
Heart patient support group, chapters, and Internet support.
www.mendedhearts.org

Grief Recovery Helpline—800-445-4808

INDEX

(Note: Italicized page numbers indicate illustrations.)

Q
Quackwatch, 296

R
Radionuclide scanning, 64–65
Recipes, 183–185
Red blood cells, 55
Regurgitation, 58
Relaxation, 143–145
The Relaxation Response, 143
Restaurants, 277
Rheumatic heart disease, 58
Risk factors, 21; age and gender, 24; care-givers', 215–216; cholesterol, 29–30; diabetes, 26–29; family history, 22–23; high blood pressure (hypertension), 25–26; high-fat diet, 32; homocysteine, 30; obesity, 31; physical inactivity, 30–31; smoking, 24–25; stress, 32–33, 45; triglycerides, 30; weight of factors, 21–22; in women, 254–262
Roizen, Michael F., 103
Role reversal, 104–107

S
Saccharin, 179
Satcher, David, 268
Self-monitoring skills, 12; breathing, 13; heartbeat, 13
Seligman, Martin E. P., 231
Senior advocates, 298
Sex: after surgery, 102–104; caregiver fear of resuming, 152–153; drug side effects, 127; and women, 261
Shakespeare, William, 52
Siebert, Al, 230
Siegel, Bernie, 230
Silver linings, 232
Simvastatin, 125
Sinoatrial node, 53
Six-point action plan, 3–5
Sleep, 159; patterns, 99
Small pleasures, 233, 235

Smoking, 24–25, 185–186; avoiding weight gain when quitting, 191; cutting back gradually, 188–189; and heart disease, 187, 188; information sources, 298; and life span, 186, 187; passive smoke, 188; preparing to quit, 188; quitting and reduction of risk, 24; and relapses, 191; supportive nonsmoking activities, 189; withdrawal symptoms, 189–191; and women, 257
Social support, 219–225
Society for Neuroscience, 149
Sodium (salt), 178
Soft drinks, 177, 269
Spiritual support, 235–239; increased chances of recovery, 236
Splenda, 179
STAR POINT 1: Take charge of your heart, 4
STAR POINT 2: Educate yourself, 4
STAR POINT 3: Lead your team, 4
STAR POINT 4: Manage your treatment, 4–5
STAR POINT 5: Live heart smart, 5
STAR POINT 6: Embrace support, 5
Stenosis, 58
Stents, 128, *128*
Stethoscopes, 60, 61
Stress, 32–33, 45, 136–137, 281; and acceptance, 147; and altering the situation, 147; and anger, 154; and avoidance, 147; in caregivers, 149; controlling, not eliminating, 141; and cutting out caffeine, 158–159; and deep breathing, 144; and exercise, 141–143; flight-or-fight response, 137; and forgiveness, 142; and fresh flowers, 144; and gardening, 142; and getting enough sleep, 159; and good nutrition, 158–159; harmful effects, 137–138; health effects, 136; and heart disease, 138–139; information source, 298; and journal writing, 141; and laughter, 148–149, 228–229; and learned optimism, 148; and learning to say no, 146; management, 138; and

ABOUT THE AUTHORS

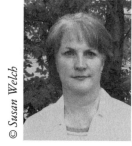

DARRELL TROUT is a writer, photographer, gardener, and lecturer. After a career in business, he became a writer and has written for magazines and completed two previous books. He had never been ill with a major illness or spent a day in the hospital until being hit with heart disease and ending up in the cardiac care unit. He began researching heart disease, treatment options, and lifestyle choices trying to figure out how to stay alive. That research helped him make decisions, change his lifestyle, and ultimately resulted in this book.

A successful educator, speaker, and author, **ELLEN WELCH** has more than 25 years' experience in the business, education, and nonprofit arenas. A former editor-in-chief of two family magazines, she has written for numerous local and national magazines and is a sought-after speaker on family and parenting issues. After Ellen's father underwent quadruple bypass surgery in August 1998, she took on a caregiver role to both her parents. Compelled to stay on top of the latest medical information to help her parents manage their health problems and to motivate herself to lead a healthy lifestyle, she understands well the critical link between caregiver, patient, and the health profession.

For information on heart disease, recent research, and support groups along with the authors' appearance schedules, check out the authors' website, **www.survivingwithheart.com.**